WELLBEING STRATEGIES

STRATEGIES

FOR NURSES

Student Survival Skills Series

Survive your nursing course with these essential guides for all student nurses:

Medicine Management Skills for Nurses, 2nd Edition
Claire Boyd
9781119807926

Clinical Skills for Nurses, 2nd Edition
Claire Boyd
9781119871545

Study Skills for Nurses
Claire Boyd
9781118657430

Care Skills for Nurses
Claire Boyd
9781118657386

Communication Skills for Nurses
Claire Boyd and Janet Dare
9781118767528

Acute Care for Nurses
Claire Boyd
9781119882459

Calculation Skills for Nurses, 2nd Edition
Claire Boyd
9781119808121

Reflective Practice for Nurses
Claire Boyd
9781119882480

WELLBEING STRATEGIES
FOR NURSES

Claire Boyd

RGN, Cert Ed
Practice Development Trainer

WILEY Blackwell

Registered Offices
John Wiley & Sons, Inc., 111 River Street, Hoboken, NJ 07030, USA
John Wiley & Sons Ltd, The Atrium, Southern Gate, Chichester, West Sussex, PO19 8SQ, UK

For details of our global editorial offices, customer services, and more information about Wiley products visit us at www.wiley.com.

Wiley also publishes its books in a variety of electronic formats and by print-on-demand. Some content that appears in standard print versions of this book may not be available in other formats.

Library of Congress Cataloging-in-Publication Data
Names: Boyd, Claire, author.
Title: Wellbeing strategies for nurses / Claire Boyd.
Other titles: Student survival skills series.
Description: Hoboken, NJ : Wiley-Blackwell, 2023. | Series: Student
  survival skills series | Includes bibliographical references and index.
Identifiers: LCCN 2022052839 (print) | LCCN 2022052840 (ebook) | ISBN
  9781119893554 (paperback) | ISBN 9781119893561 (adobe pdf) | ISBN
  9781119893578 (epub)
Subjects: MESH: Nurses–psychology | Self Care | Relaxation
  Therapy–methods | Mindfulness
Classification: LCC RT41 (print) | LCC RT41 (ebook) | NLM WY 87 | DDC
  610.73–dc23/eng/20230120
LC record available at https://lccn.loc.gov/2022052839
LC ebook record available at https://lccn.loc.gov/2022052840

Cover Design: Wiley
Cover Images: © Media Manager; Wiley; ohaiyoo/Adobe Stock Photos; Vaclav Krivsky/Shutterstock

Set in Trade Gothic Light 9/12pt by Straive, Pondicherry, India
Printed and bound by CPI Group (UK) Ltd, Croydon, CR0 4YY

C9781119893554_010323

Contents

PART 3 Guided Meditation for Groups and Individuals 255

Preface

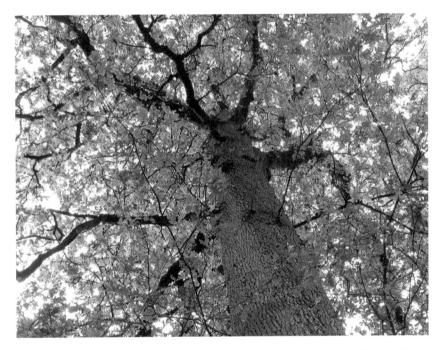

As healthcare professionals, we look after the wellbeing of our patients/clients. This book is about looking after *you*, the carer. With nurses leaving the profession in record numbers, often citing stress and burnout as contributing factors, this book is a vital addition to the other books in the student survival series.

This book looks at wellbeing strategies used in healthcare, education, business and many other sectors due to the 'duty of care' philosophy.

There are over 180 exercises and activities for the individual so you can dip your toes in and find the ones that work for you. As with other books in the series, this book has been divided into sections, with Part Three designed for groups if you wish to get together with colleagues and friends for a more in-depth wellbeing session.

All these strategies have been practised on student nurses, nursing associates, registered nurses and midwives, and other healthcare staff and have been adapted for optimum enjoyment.

Keep in mind: if you feel overwhelmed with stress, please see a professional, sooner rather than later.

Introduction

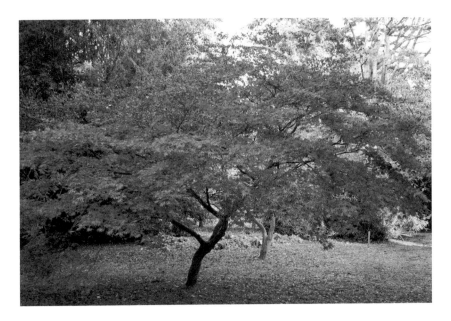

There is no job on earth quite like the nursing/caring profession. It has been a huge privilege to nurse patients back to health and even at times to facilitate a dignified and comfortable death.

After caring for patients, it has never ceased to amaze me when patients who have been discharged send me a 'thank you' letter – not because I thought my care was poor, but because they took the time and trouble to do this! A little kindness goes a long way.

Now to take off the rose-tinted spectacles: there have also been times in my nursing career when I went home in tears because of my frustration with my heavy workload and inability to provide the care I came into the profession to deliver to my patients. This sub-optimal care was, to be honest, just fire-fighting: for example, covering for colleagues due to sickness and understaffing issues, working many extra unpaid hours, and being so exhausted that when I eventually arrived home, I was too tired to eat the lovely supper my family had prepared for me. Working in neurosciences, I also had to contend with the occasional patients with steroid-induced psychosis throwing chairs and punches towards me. In short, working in healthcare can be mega-stressful!

As a healthcare professional working for the NHS and in the healthcare sector for 40 years, I am used to dealing with these pressures and 'winter pressures' when wards are full and ambulances are stacked outside A & E with patients waiting to be admitted with the flu virus, chest infections, and an increase in slips and falls due to slippery pavements. But the last few years have been like no other time in health-care – staff fatigue and exhaustion have taken on a whole new dimension because of the coronavirus pandemic. Only today, a colleague told me that working in these conditions is 'soul destroying'. You can only run on empty for so long before the wheels come off. Healthcare professionals now need the care and kindness we are so used to giving to others.

As a nurse and a holistic therapist, I prepare relaxation sessions for my stressed colleagues, using beautiful pictures of nature to gaze into, beautiful smells to bring joy, lovely foods to evoke happiness, breathing exercises to relieve stress, mindful-ness to slow down our frantic pace of life, humour to initiate the 'happy hormones' (e.g. Serotonin) and meditation and visualisations to take us to beautiful settings in our mind's eye.

This book uses all these strategies I use during my sessions. If you only want to use the guided visualisation scripts, you will need someone to read the words to you, or you can record them yourself on your phone and play them back when you have some 'me time'. This time is not a luxury; it is vital for your wellbeing, just like eating and drinking.

Perhaps you would like to use some of the smaller exercises and tips for relieving stress, like using essential oils or mindfulness. Perhaps you want to go the whole hog and prepare an entire session, including dressing the room – such as laying out shells and exotic fruits for the tropical paradise session. Each seasonal guided visualisation session takes about 40–50 minutes (or less time, if you wish).

You do not have to be a trained therapist in any of the therapies in this book, as I have chosen safe exercises for the layperson to enjoy. For example, you will not be putting essential oils on the skin to massage, so you do not need to know the science of the oils or contraindications or even how the oil was obtained (steam, expression, etc.).

Just as a postscript, there are many 'New Age' books on the market with some dubious claims. This book only looks at accepted wellbeing strategies used in healthcare. However, if stripping off nude and rolling in long grass and nettles covered in morning dew works for you, then carry on! (Apparently this is a real thing in parts of Scandinavia – no judgements here!)

Take from this book whatever you need.

As with other books in the series, this book comes in three parts:

Part One looks at stress and what it does to our bodies, and why strategies for self-care are so important. We will also look at why shift work can disrupt our natural sleeping patterns and how we can counteract this.

Part Two looks at 13 strategies to combat stress. We discuss each in a no-nonsense way and give you the important information – what you need to know without all the fluff, keeping it short and snappy.

Part Three consists of guided meditation exercises using seasonal themes, such as a tropical paradise and a walk in the snow. I will show you how to dress a room for larger groups or use the visualisation exercises just for you. All these exercises have been used by healthcare workers who have enjoyed the experiences and helped me adapt the sessions for the perfect relaxation experience. Like other books in this series, this book has been developed for the healthcare worker by healthcare workers who have given me tips and guidance for each of the strategies. For example, during an earlier version of the meadow guided meditation script, I talked about 'listening to the distant croaks of the frogs in the long grass'. Afterwards, one of my colleagues told me that she has a phobia of toads and frogs, and this made her anxious, destroying her enjoyment of the session. Needless to say, all mention of frogs and toads was removed from the script!

Other books in this series have a "Test Your Knowledge" section at the end of each chapter. This book has an activity related to the chapter contents – something for you to enjoy. There are also little exercises to dip your toes into the therapies. Find what works for you. For me, you can't beat a sprinkling of all the therapies in one session.

Let me tell you about some lovely Filipino nurses I once had the pleasure of working with. First, you need to imagine the sense of wonder of seeing snow for the first time ever; they were delighted to see a blanket of white across the hospital grounds and rushed to put on their coats and go out and hear the crunch beneath their feet. It seemed unkind to inform them that this was, in fact, just a heavy frost. When it did actually snow, you could hear their shrieks of joy for miles! When was the last time you experienced such happiness?

Please take time to care for yourself. Remember, care begins with self-care. And if you are struggling, seek professional help for your wellbeing.

Acknowledgements

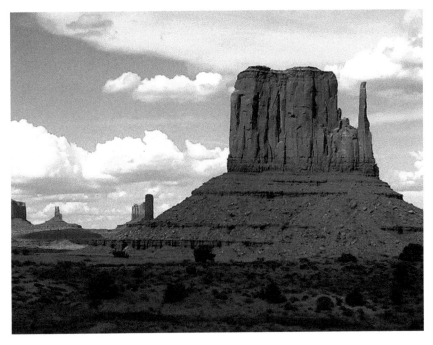

Thanks go firstly to my work colleagues at North Bristol Healthcare Trust, including the student nurses and nurse associates who attended the relaxation sessions I prepared – how we enjoyed floating on a cloud and wiggling like seaweed on our yoga mats! How we also enjoyed all the lovely places we visited in our imagination. Happy days! Thanks for all the encouragement to share this book with a wider audience.

ACKNOWLEDGEMENTS

Thanks also go to Rob, my lovely husband and soul mate, for the beautiful photos. And to my son Simon, who, years ago, when I was studying for my diploma in thermal-auricular therapy (ear candling) and before I had a treatment couch, fell asleep on the floor after the treatment; we left you for a couple of hours and just stepped over you while going about our day! Thanks also to Owen and Rhys (my fantastic grandsons), who allow me to practice some of my techniques on them!

Thanks also to all at Wiley who helped bring this series of books to fruition.

This book is dedicated to all the NHS and community carers and the vital keyworkers who kept and continue to keep the country running during times of lockdown and pandemic. Enjoy!

PART 1

· · · · · · · · · · · · · · · · · · · ·

OCCUPATIONAL ILL-HEALTH

Stress

Anxiety

PTSD

Compassion Fatigue

Burnout

Wellbeing Strategies for Nurses, First Edition. Claire Boyd.
© 2023 John Wiley & Sons Ltd. Published 2023 by John Wiley & Sons Ltd.

Chapter 1

SELF-CARE AND WELLBEING

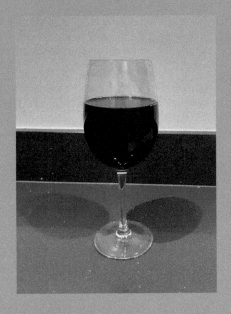

LEARNING OUTCOMES

By the end of this chapter, you will have an understanding of the importance of self-care and wellbeing in healthcare to help with compassion fatigue, burnout, and post-traumatic stress disorder.

Different approaches to wellbeing techniques will be explored, including acupuncture, acupressure, yoga, Qigong, Tai Chi, and massage.

How are you feeling today? I ask this because we know the NHS is in a 'jobs crisis' with large numbers of healthcare professionals in the UK leaving the profession, citing as their reasons for leaving 'pay, working conditions and feeling under huge pressure'. Those leaving the profession often are not replaced, and the shortfall of healthcare professionals is reaching record levels, which puts more pressure on those still hanging on and caring for the vulnerable.

But who is looking after you? We do need to look after ourselves, as laid out by the Nursing & Midwifery Council document 'Future Nurse: Standards of Proficiency for Registered Nurses' (2018). This document states that at the point of registration, the nurse will:

1.5   understand the demands of professional practice and demonstrate how to recognise signs of vulnerability in themselves or their colleagues and the action required to minimize risks to health
1.6   understand the professional responsibility to adopt a healthy lifestyle to maintain the level of personal fitness and wellbeing required to meet people's needs for mental and physical care.

In short, it is all about self-care and wellbeing. We need to care for ourselves and our colleagues, which may be easier said than done in today's healthcare climate.

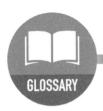

GLOSSARY

Self-care
The actions we take for ourselves to remain fit and healthy and understand when we can look after ourselves and when we need to seek help from other healthcare professionals.

Wellbeing
Represents a broader bio-psycho-social construct that includes physical, mental, and social health.

The self-care process can start by reflecting on what makes us happy. When we are going through trying times, it can be easy to focus on the negative aspects of our lives – causing us even more stress and anxiety. Before we go down a negative spiral, it is important to focus on the things that make us happy. Moving from the negative to the positive is an important aspect of the healing process. And note that we may need help with this process (counselling, general practitioners, etc.).

COMPASSION FATIGUE

Unique to the healthcare sector is the occupational stressor known as **compassion fatigue**, whereby the carer connects with a patient and feels how they are feeling. This opens them up to absorbing and experiencing the patient's trauma, suffering, and pain – known as **vicarious traumatisation**. This exposure stimulates our fight-or-flight response, which we then continually suppress, leading to consequences for our physical and mental health.

The symptoms of compassion fatigue can be seen in Table 1.1.

If we ignore the body's response to vicarious trauma, the physical symptoms will only get worse. This is when we need

Table 1.1 Symptoms of compassion fatigue.

Phase 1	Anxiety	Vicarious trauma stimulates the nervous system into flight or fight, and you feel the effects of adrenaline on the body – raised heart and breathing rates, shaking, and muscle tension. It becomes harder to think clearly and concentrate and may be harder to sleep. It becomes more difficult to relax.
Phase 2	Irritability	Chronic stress may induce headaches, fatigue, and multiple minor illnesses as the immune system becomes compromised. The tension may affect your musculoskeletal system, causing chronic neck and back pain. You may eat more (or less) than usual.
Phase 3	Withdrawal	As you experience chronic fatigue and constant aches and pains, you may start to neglect your physical and emotional health. If you take time off from work, you do not feel any better on your return.
Phase 4	Robot	These symptoms are very similar to those suffering from depression and also include headaches, generalised aches and pains, digestive problems, and a feeling of low-level anxiety and very low mood.

to take steps to care for ourselves before we experience burnout.

BURNOUT

Burnout is a syndrome resulting from chronic workplace stress that has not been successfully managed. It is characterised by three dimensions:

1 Feelings of energy depletion or exhaustion
2 Increased mental distance from one's job or feelings of negativism or cynicism related to one's job
3 Reduced professional efficacy

Risk factors associated with increased susceptibility to developing Burnout Syndrome can be seen in Table 1.2.

Table 1.3 shows some of the actions we can take to prevent Burnout Syndrome in the workplace.

Table 1.2 Risk factors in developing Burnout Syndrome.

Individual risk factors	• Poor self-esteem • Poor coping strategies • Idealistic world view • Unrealistically high expectations • Financial issues
Organisational risk factors	• Heavy workload • Conflicts with co-workers • Diminished resources • Lack of control or input • Effort-reward imbalance • Understaffing • Rapid institutional changes
Risk factors for nurses	• Variability in work schedules • Rapid turnover of patients • End-of-life events • No breaks during shifts

Table 1.3 Action steps to prevent Burnout Syndrome.

Manage	Understand that there are ways in which you can manage your work-related stressors that put you at risk of Burnout Syndrome.
Engage	Engage in the support of management, co-workers, friends, and family that may help you cope with stress – this is not a weakness.
Breaks	Take breaks at work and away from work. Go outside for a walk to get some fresh air during your breaks.
Enjoyment	Think about what you enjoy about your work, and focus your attention on your interests and passions.
Techniques	Gain techniques to be used at work when dealing with stressful work experiences and after work to relax and recharge.

STRESS-RELIEVING STRATEGIES

To effectively combat stress, we need to activate the body's natural relaxation response. We are all unique human beings, and stress-relieving strategies are not a case of 'one size fits all'. Each of us has preferred calming stress busters. The following bullet points show some of the strategies you may utilise to reach a state of calm and unwind after a stressful day or on a day off:

- Spending a day at a spa
- Eating chocolate
- Drinking a glass of wine at the end of the day
- Taking a walk in the country
- Going for a swim
- Going to the hairdresser/having your hair washed
- Going for a run
- Meditating
- Going somewhere for quiet time (stillness)
- Going to the gym
- Reading a book
- Undertaking some arts and crafts (hobbies)
- Watching a movie
- Listening to music
- Going to a café for a hot beverage (and a piece of cake) with friends
- Soaking in a warm bath
- Having a massage
- Gardening
- Playing with your pet animal
- Watching a football/rugby match (could be stressful if your team lose)
- Doing yoga
- Working on a jigsaw puzzle
- Modelling with LEGO bricks

I live in the West of England, and one of my favourite ways to destress is to go for a short walk in the Cotswold countryside and then stop in an Olde Worlde tea shop for a cup of tea and some cream scones (jam first, cream on top). Sometimes I forego the walk! (Several of my colleagues like to go to the gym after work – I can't think of anything worse!) My husband likes to snuggle up on the settee with a hot cup of tea, dunking his biscuits (yuk!) whilst watching a good movie on Netflix. In other words, it really is horses for courses. Also, everything in moderation: we should not become dependent on pouring alcohol down our gullets to 'feel better' as this could be a slippery slope.

The important thing is that we all need an outlet for our stress. Good health relies not just on the physical aspect but also the mental health aspect – a truly holistic approach. Also, if money is an issue, as it is for most of us, unless you can dip in the sea or go in for wild swimming in the local riverways, paying to swim in the local swimming pool or visiting the hairdresser frequently may be impractical due to cost.

Making 'Me Time'

Sometimes we may feel we don't have enough hours for such luxuries as 'me time' because work and life encroach on our precious days. When we are not at work, we may have family life to contend with, washing, shopping and cooking, or simply catching up on sleep due to exhaustion. Perhaps we also have assignments to complete. Believing we can't spare a little time for self-care is a false economy. You can't run a car on fumes; the car requires refuelling when almost empty, just like the body needs calm time to combat stress. You take medicine for a headache, so why not take medicine for the soul, as stress-relief strategies are often called? Caring for your mental health is not a luxury. Using the car analogy again, if the engine breaks down, the car won't work. If the body is struggling due to stress, you won't be efficient in your work or personal life.

EXERCISE 1.1 Yoghurt Mask

Spending a little time for yourself need not cost a fortune. A nice pampering exercise if you have a little plain yoghurt left over is to use it as a face mask, which will leave your skin feeling refreshed and smooth. Remember to put some old towels under your head on the pillow for spillage!

One of the most beneficial substances to use as a face pack is yoghurt (live, natural yoghurt, full-fat if possible). Fresh, live yoghurt can help all skin types, particularly excessively dry or oily skin. The lactic acid in yoghurt (due to its fermentation) is similar to that of the skin acid mantle and appears to exert a balancing action on the secretions of skin fluids.

Add mashed-up banana, papaya, or any over-ripe fruit of your choice to two teaspoons of yoghurt. Rub the mixture into your face. Relax. You may wish to put two cucumber slices on your eyes (to reduce puffiness). Rinse off with plenty of water.

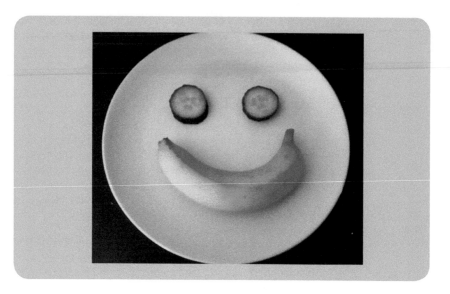

Healthcare Stress

We have already seen how working in healthcare can be extremely stressful. In the first quarter of the twenty-first century, the world was introduced to the coronavirus pandemic, and healthcare workers were hailed as heroes for caring for unprecedented numbers of patients with the virus. Many worked extra shifts to cover for colleagues isolating with the virus or on sick leave, perhaps due to sheer exhaustion. We also needed to care for patients – the death and grief of the patients who knew they were dying. We are not robots, so these sad memories will stay with us forever. Caring for the carer has never been so important.

DID YOU KNOW?

One in nine health staff left the NHS during the coronavirus pandemic – and the exodus is speeding up, according to official figures (2022). 140 000 workers quit amid the crisis, and according to staff surveys, another 31% are thinking of leaving. Exhaustion, low pay, and stress were cited as reasons for this exodus. Unison's Christina McAnea states that staff are suffering from exhaustion, burnout and PTSD in some cases (https://www.pressreader.com/uk/sunday-mirr or/20220424/281582359187651).

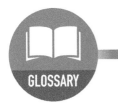

GLOSSARY

PTSD
Post-traumatic stress disorder. A mental health condition that develops following a traumatic event, characterised by intrusive thoughts about the incident, recurrent distress/anxiety, flashbacks, and avoidance of similar situations.

RELAXATION TECHNIQUES

It is safe to say that finding a strategy for stress relief has never been so important. It is really just finding the strategy that works for you. Roughly speaking, the most popular approaches can be grouped into seven main categories, as shown in Table 1.4. We will look at each of the examples throughout this book and/or in this chapter.

Table 1.4 Seven tactics for stress relief.

Tactic 1	Focus your mind to bring about the relaxation response.	Examples: Deep breathing (Chapter 4) Meditation (Chapter 12) Mindfulness (Chapter 13) Progressive muscle relaxation (Chapter 5)
Tactic 2	Redefine the situation mentally so that it is no longer viewed as a threatening situation.	Examples: Humour (Chapter 11) Imagery (Chapter 14)
Tactic 3	Use Eastern methods to restore your mental and physical balance.	Example: Acupressure (Chapter 2)
Tactic 4	Use yoga/yoga breathing to calm the mind and relax the body.	Examples: Yoga breathing (Chapter 2) Yoga (Chapter 2)
Tactic 5	Relieve muscle tension through exercise and massage.	Examples: Stretching (Chapter 2) Massage (Chapter 1) Physical exercise (Chapter 7)

(Continued)

Table 1.4 (*Continued*)

Tactic 6	Fill your mind with thoughts of pleasure rather than threats.	Examples: Aromatherapy (Chapter 9) Music (Chapter 15) Nature (Chapter 6) Social support (Chapter 10)
Tactic 7	Use coping strategies for stress before stress becomes a problem.	Examples: Eating well (Chapter 7) Hydrating well (Chapter 7) Sleeping well (Chapter 3)

Overthinking

Even the most chilled of us get stressed at times – going over and over a situation in our mind and being unable to shake off these thoughts. Perhaps we had a difficult shift or received harsh feedback from an assignment or the placement we are on. These thoughts may make us anxious and lead to depression over time. But we can do something about it.

Stop and rethink: Going over the same negative situation again and again is not healthy. Look for the positives instead of concentrating on the negatives, no matter how small you think they are. Many people have told me that when a family member became ill, it put all their stress and anxieties about other things into perspective.

Example: *spoke harshly to my colleague and feel bad about this. I can't stop feeling upset about this.*

Finding the positive: *With hindsight, I now believe that I did not speak over-harshly, and she does need to concentrate on the task in hand for patient safety. I did the right thing.*

Make time to worry: Set aside some time to write down all your worries. Then work through the list to find solutions to the problems you can control and let go of the things you can't control.

Example: Can't afford to pay all my bills this month. Speak to the bank about extending my overdraft.

Did not get the promotion I went for. Let this go as I was too good for them. Look out for other Band 6 positions and work on my interview skills.

Seek help: If you feel you can't find a solution to your worries, never hesitate to seek help.

Examples:

If you worry about your job – speak to your manager.

If you worry about your mental health – speak to your GP or workplace counsellor.

If you worry about money – speak to your bank and/or Union, who have financial advisers.

Remember to speak to your colleagues, friends, family, and professionals – do not suffer alone.

If you feel your negative thoughts are becoming overwhelming, cognitive behavioural therapy (CBT) can help to reframe your negative thoughts, enabling you to cope with your anxiety.

STUDENT TIP

As a first-year student, I once worked with a third-year student who just didn't like me. That's fine as we can't get along with everyone. Instead of going over and over thinking about what I was doing to make her dislike me so much, I turned this around and realised that the problem was actually hers, which helped to relieve my stress. I was always polite and professional to her. The last I heard, she left the nursing profession – some people just aren't cut out to be kind and compassionate.

Taking Control

If you ever think 'I can't do anything about my problem', your stress will inevitably get worse, as this feeling of loss of control is one of the main causes of stress and lack of wellbeing. Taking control is empowering and a crucial part of finding a solution.

However, you need to accept the things you can't change, as changing a difficult situation is not always possible. It is therefore important to concentrate on the things you have control over.

Research in Treating Anxiety and Psychological Disorders

Anxiety and psychological disorders affect 264 million people worldwide. Unfortunately, anti-anxiety medications aren't effective for everyone, and many of these drugs have unwanted side effects. As a means of understanding the brain networks and mechanisms that underlie fear and anxiety and hopefully offering a new and better approach to treatments, Bristol University researchers have been studying the brain's cerebellum. The cerebellum is connected to many regions of the brain that are linked to survival, including the PAG (periaqueductal grey).

TERMINOLOGY

The **periaqueductal grey** is a structure in the brain that coordinates survival mechanisms, including the 'freezing' behaviour when we feel paralysed with fear.

Researchers have found that the PAG can form a 'fear memory' when fear is felt, accompanied by freezing, meaning the cerebellum encodes a fear memory that returns and replays (think post-traumatic stress). The Bristol University researchers have shown that manipulating the cerebellar-PAG pathway can lessen fear-conditioned freezing in animals.

The Bristol University Researchers explain:

> Our results show that the cerebellum is part of the brain's survival network that regulates fear memory processes at multiple timescales and in multiple ways, raising the possibility that dysfunctional interactions in the brain's cerebellar-survival network may underlie fear-related disorders and co-morbidities. (www.mirror.co.uk/lifestyle/health/hope-scientists-targeting-new-area-26970056)

This has radically changed our way of thinking about anxiety. Previously, we believed anxiety was generated in deep brain centres such as the amygdala and in response to stress hormones. Finding this other site for anxiety in the cerebellum gives a whole new approach for drugs and therapies, targeting new ways of treating psychological conditions such as PTSD.

EXERCISE 1.2   Melting the Ice Sculpture

This is a good exercise to help release the anxieties and tension that lead to stress:

1   Close your eyes and imagine a beautiful ice sculpture of a swan in front of you.
2   Mentally list anything in your life that is causing stress: at work, at home, anywhere.
3   Each time you think of something, say it out loud. Imagine that as you say it, a warm gust of air travels towards the ice swan, and the sculpture begins to melt.
4   Continue venting all your worries and watching the swan melt before you.
5   Soon all your worries have turned the swan into a crystal clear puddle of water, taking all your stress with it.

DID YOU KNOW?

The Japanese have invented a 'scream jar'. This is a handheld jar that you can scream into to let out all your stress. You put the jar neck up to your mouth and literally scream into it. It is soundproofed, so you may only hear a faint whisper.

Learning New Skills

Learning some simple yoga poses may help with stress levels in ways we did not know previously. Research has shown that learning new skills can improve your mental wellbeing by:

- Boosting self-confidence and raising self-esteem
- Helping to build a sense of purpose
- Helping you connect with others

Even if we feel we do not have time or do not need to learn new things, there are many ways we can incorporate this into our lives, such as:

- Learning to cook something new
- Working on a DIY project (something we have been meaning to fix for a while)
- Signing up for a course that interests us, such as learning a new language
- Signing up for a class in something we have always wanted to learn, like Salsa dancing or yoga
- Taking up a new hobby

LOOKING AT THE EASTERN APPROACH

There are many Eastern approaches to healthcare, some of which you may have heard of and others not: Qigong, Tai Chi, feng shui, acupressure, reiki, shiatsu, and yoga, to name just a few. We shall look at four of these: Qigong, Tai Chi, acupressure, and yoga and yoga breathing.

Eastern approaches to healthcare include methods for relieving stress by restoring mental and physical balance. The basic belief of the Eastern approach is that stress, disease, and injury disrupt the vital energy inside the body, whilst meditation, breathing exercises, movement, and massage help to restore it.

Acupuncture and Acupressure

Acupuncture has long been used within the NHS to treat conditions such as pain, hypertension, insomnia, stress, depression, etc. Acupuncture uses needles that are placed along the body's meridians, known as acupoints.

TERMINOLOGY

Meridians: Channels that direct the flow of energy through specific pathways of the body, much like the circulatory system transports blood around the body.

Another technique using acupoints is acupressure. Acupressure practitioners stimulate the acupoints using fingers or other tools. As with acupuncture, each point is said to affect particular organs or tissues of the body. Most scientific studies have concentrated on needle acupuncture, but acupressure without needles has also been found to affect health and wellbeing.

A 2002 report by the World Health Organisation (WHO) listed 28 diseases, symptoms, and conditions for which acupuncture, in controlled trials, was shown to be an effective treatment. A further 63 trials showed favourable results, but further trials were recommended.

It is still not known exactly how acupressure works, but scientists have sought to explain it:

- It is simply a relaxing form of massage.
- A report from the United States (section of the National Institutes of Health – National Centre for complementary and alternative medicines) states that acupuncture points may be strategic conductors of electromagnetic signals. Stimulating the meridians may enable electromagnetic signals within the body to be relayed at a faster rate than normal. These signals may cause the release of brain chemicals (such as endorphins, etc.) that reduce pain sensations and feelings of wellbeing. This may also activate the immune system.

EXERCISE 1.3 Acupressure

The acupressure point for stress is located on the ear. Try this technique and see if it works for you:

1   Remove any jewellery from the ear. Do not try this exercise if your ears are sore or infected, obviously! Close your eyes, and grasp both earlobes between your thumbs and index fingers. Gently squeeze and pull the lobes downward. Take three deep breaths.

2   Move your thumbs and fingers a little higher up the outer edge of the earlobe. Lightly pinch, holding for a few seconds. Continue moving all the way up the outside of the ear: i.e. pinch and hold and move upward.

3   When you get to the top of the ears, gently squeeze and pull the ears upward. Take three deep breaths.

4   To finish, lightly cup your ears with your hands.

YOGA

The word **yoga** may conjure in your mind an image of a person in impossible poses. Whilst it is true that there are many different styles of yoga varying in intensity and focus, some aspects of this ancient practice can be quite easy to follow. Yoga brings together the mind and the body, using **focussed breathing** exercises, **meditation**, and **physical poses** designed to encourage relaxation and reduce stress. We will look at a focused breathing exercise, a typical yoga breathing meditation, and a couple of easy-to-perform poses. But first, Table 1.5 shows 16 benefits of yoga that are supported by scientific evidence:

Table 1.5 16 benefits of yoga.

1. Yoga improves flexibility.	Flexibility is an important component of physical health. Yoga offers many styles to choose from, varying in intensity from high to moderate to mild. Even the lowest-intensity styles have been found to increase flexibility.
2. Yoga helps with stress relief.	Scientific research supports that yoga can reduce stress, but we need to remember that the physical practice is only one aspect of yoga. Other aspects of yoga, such as meditation and breath work, have also been shown to significantly lessen tension and relieve stress.
3. Yoga improves mental health.	Both movement-based yoga therapies and breathing-based practices have been shown to significantly improve depressive symptoms and other mental health disorders.
4. Yoga may reduce inflammation.	Research studies have found that yoga of various styles, intensities, and durations can reduce the biochemical markers of inflammation across several chronic conditions.
5. Yoga can increase strength.	Studies have shown that some types of yoga can be considered strength-building.
6. Yoga may reduce anxiety.	The yoga practice of body scan/guided meditation has been shown to reduce symptoms of anxiety.
7. Yoga may improve quality of life.	A study in 2019 showed a promising potential for yoga to improve quality of life (as defined by the WHO) in people with chronic pain.

(Continued)

Table 1.5 (*Continued*)

8. Yoga may improve immunity.	Chronic stress negatively affects the immune system. Some studies have found a link between practising yoga and better immune system functioning.
9. Yoga may improve cardiovascular functioning.	Yoga breathing can improve the functioning of several systems in the body. By controlling the pace of breathing, the cardiovascular system can make favourable changes in heart rate, stroke capacity, arterial pressure, and contractility of the heart.
10. Yoga may improve sleep.	Yoga has been shown to improve how quickly someone falls asleep and how deeply they stay asleep.
11. Yoga may improve self-esteem.	Studies have shown positive results when using yoga to improve self-esteem and perceived body image in adolescents and young adults.
12. Yoga may improve bone health.	Many postures in yoga are isometric contractions (the length of the muscles holding a pose does not change, although they are fully engaged). These isometric exercises, especially when performed with the joints in flexion, have been found to increase bone density, although more studies need to be performed.
13. Yoga can promote better posture and body awareness.	Studies have found that yoga improved brain functioning in the centres responsible for interception (recognising the sensations within your body) and better posture.
14. Yoga can improve brain functioning.	Practising yoga has been found to activate areas of the brain responsible for motivation, executive functioning, attention, and neuroplasticity.
15. Yoga can help with burnout.	Studies have found that yoga-based meditation interventions can reduce the effects of burnout as individuals become more in-tune with and more likely to listen to their body's signals and respond appropriately.
16. Yoga can improve balance.	Falls in healthcare facilities can lead to decreased quality of life in individuals and even death in some cases. Research suggests that balance may improve for most people after consistently practising yoga.

Yoga Breathing

Breathing techniques play a large role in many relaxation techniques, so it is little wonder that focused breathing is such an important aspect of yoga. We will look at different breathing techniques in more depth in Chapter 4. But let's try the cooling breath technique (known as Sitkari Pranayama), so-called due to its effects, when practised correctly, of calming and 'cooling' the nervous system, combatting stress and anxiety.

EXERCISE 1.4   The Cooling Breath

1   Sit comfortably on the floor or a chair, ensuring that the spine is erect with a natural curve and relaxing the shoulders.
2   Open your mouth slightly, and place your tongue gently behind your top teeth.
3   Inhale through your mouth as you raise your chin.
4   Close your mouth, and exhale through your nose as you lower your chin to a neutral position.
5   Repeat 8–12 times.

Yoga Meditation Breathing Script

This next exercise is a typical yoga meditation breathing script.

EXERCISE 1.5   Meditation Breathing Script

1   Sit or lie in a comfortable position, and give yourself permission to relax and unwind.
2   Just sit quietly for 2–10 minutes.
3   Close your eyes. Turn your attention to your everyday breath, and listen to the sound and movement as it flows softly in and out through your nose.
4   On your next breath, slowly breathe in and quietly count 'One'.
5   Breathe out, and count 'Two'.

6   Breathe in, and count 'Three'.

7   Breathe out, and count 'Four'. Continue counting your breaths up to 10.

8   When you reach the number 10, go back to 1 and repeat the practice for 2–10 minutes.

9   If your mind wanders during the practice and you lose concentration, return your attention to your breath and begin counting from one.

10   When you are ready, slowly open your eyes and enjoy the feeling of calm for a moment.

Note that you do not have to sit in the cross-legged yoga position to perform this exercise – unless you want to, of course!

Yoga Poses (for the Beginner)

Muscle tension is often a side effect of stress. Stretching can loosen the muscles, which can help with aches, pains, and stiffness and help to relax the mind. Don't be put off by these poses; they are designed for yoga beginners. Even I can do them without needing a hoist to get me back to a standing position!

One very simple pose is the Easy Seated Pose, another name for sitting cross-legged. Get seated in a cross-legged position – with practice, you can try to keep your feet directly below your knees. Keep your hands on your knees or lap, and try to keep your back straight. Don't hunch over or keep your head down.

EXERCISE 1.6   Yoga Poses for Beginners

Cat pose	This pose is good for giving your back a good stretch.	Get on all fours, and then push your palms down as you 'round' your back. Keep your head down and your arms straight, and hold this pose. Basically, you want to keep your back curved like a bow (as in bow and arrow).

Cobra pose

This pose is also known as an upward-facing dog and is good for stretching your back.

Lie on your stomach with your feet slightly apart, placing your palms directly under your shoulders. Pull your chest forward and up, creating a deep backbend and lengthening your tailbone.

Bridge pose

This pose is also good for strengthening your back.

Lie on your back with your arms at your sides and your legs bent. Then lift your hips. Hold your body in this position for a few breaths. Keep your feet planted close to your hips.

Mountain pose

This is a standing pose and helps to keep your body aligned.

Stand with your legs together or hip-length apart. Keep your shoulders pushed down and away from your ears. Make sure your back is straight. You want to lengthen up through your spine. Your arms should be at your sides with your palms up.

Tree pose

This pose strengthens the muscles in the legs and improves ankle and thigh strength.

One foot is planted on the ground. Your other foot should slide up your inner thigh or calf. Your hands go upward in a prayer-like motion.

Corpse pose

Holding this pose requires mental concentration. It is usually performed by expert yoga practitioners at the end of a more physical workout.

You literally just lie flat on your back, keeping your arms to your sides. You can cover yourself with a blanket to keep warm.

DID YOU KNOW?

A recent study linked the ability to balance on one leg for 10 seconds with life expectancy. The test, known as the Flamingo test, found that middle-aged people who cannot balance on one leg for 10 seconds are at a dramatically increased risk of dying within seven years. To conduct the test, you need to:

1. Take off your shoes.
2. Put your hands on your hips and stand on one leg, bringing your other leg halfway up your calf.
3. See how long you last.

Failure to perform the task for 10 seconds could indicate a possible neurological or orthopaedic disorder, weight gain, inactivity, inner ear issues, or too little sleep or exhaustion. Interventions could then be implemented to prolong life.
You can improve your balance with activities such as yoga.

QIGONG

Qigong was developed in ancient China and Tibet and is a mind-body exercise form that uses meditation, breathing, and movement. It is often practised outside in parks and performed in silence. Basically, it consists of movements that you perform for certain situations, such as stress relief or to 'open the lungs'.

There are many Qigong exercises, but a simple one is called 'Bouncing on heels to shake off stress and illness' (not a very snappy title)! This exercise stimulates the immune system and removes stress and illness from the body whilst promoting clarity and increasing energy.

EXERCISE 1.7   Bouncing on Heels to Shake Off Stress and Illness

You will need to breathe deeply and slowly throughout the exercise:

1   Stand flat-footed with your heels together and toes apart in a V formation.
2   Breathe in and raise your palms upward as you bend your knees.
3   Breathe out as you push your hands towards the floor, straighten your legs, and rise up onto your tip-toes. Hold for three seconds.
4   Bounce on your heels seven times in a relaxed, natural way. On the eighth bounce, stand flat-footed and shake your body eight times.
5   Bend your knees up and down whilst throwing your arms down.
6   Repeat all these movements from the start eight times.

TAI CHI

Tai Chi is another ancient Chinese exercise form. It is a series of movements that work on the entire body in a flowing sequence – often described as meditation in motion. Tai Chi is believed to reduce stress and anxiety and help increase flexibility and balance. One very simple exercise that can be performed almost anywhere is the 'pouring' exercise.

EXERCISE 1.8   Pouring Exercise

1   Stand with your feet on the floor, parallel, shoulder-width apart.
2   Pour your weight onto one leg and hold.
3   After a few breaths in and out, begin to slowly pour your body weight onto the other leg and hold.
4   Do this for a few minutes, clearing your mind and becoming aware of your balance.

BODY MASSAGE

Massage is the application of pressure to the soft tissues of the body, such as the skin, muscles, tendons, and ligaments. The general purpose of massage is to reduce tension and stress, improve blood and lymphatic circulation, and remove toxins. It also reduces oedema, aids healing of soft-tissue injuries, controls pain, and promotes overall wellbeing by releasing endorphins.

Massage may therefore be used to relax or invigorate, depending on your needs and level of stress and the techniques used: e.g. effleurage for a soothing effect on sensory nerves and relaxing contracted, tense muscles to induce **relaxation**, or **atonement** to tone muscles and stimulate sensory nerve endings.

In clinical trials, massage has been found to relieve anxiety and depression and improve health in other areas, such as easing back pain and labour pain. Massage can therefore be shown to have a role in the 'stress war'. It is suggested that to benefit fully from the beneficial effects of massage, you should seek out a professional massage therapist, but we may not all have access to a professional masseuse, perhaps due to financial constraints. Therefore the next exercise shows how to give a very basic back massage without essential oils (just a commercial massage cream or oil). All you need is a willing partner or friend and a very light touch. A quick word of caution: only perform a massage on someone without any underlying medical conditions (leave that to the professionals).

EXERCISE 1.9   How to Give a Basic Back Massage

1   Choose a comfortable location (massage couch, bed, or floor).
2   Put down a soft mat, such as a yoga mat, and spread a clean towel over it.
3   Prepare the room (subdued lighting, aromatherapy candles, ambient music and a warm temperature).
4   Have the person expose their back and lie face down. Make a horse-shoe shape with a towel for them to place their face on. To support the individual's lower back, put a cushion beneath their ankles.
5   Tell the person you are about to begin, and remind them to take a slow deep breath to help with their relaxation.

6   Put massage oil in the palms of your clean hands.

7   Spread the oil on the back using the whole of your hands, starting at the bottom of the person's back and moving in an upward direction towards the heart whilst applying light pressure. Then bring the hands down the outside of the back, again lightly. This is known as **effleurage**.

8   Repeat this technique for three to five minutes whilst gradually increasing from light to medium pressure – this will warm the back muscles.

9   Now for the shoulder and neck area: use shorter circular strokes with more pressure – a technique that uses rolling and pressing. This is known as **petrissage**. Go across the entire back for two to five minutes.

10 Cup your hands and make brief, repetitive contacts with the back. This is known as **percussion**.

11 Use muscle-lifting techniques by making a lobster-claw shape with your hands (close your fingers and hold out the thumb).

12 Apply pressure in a twisting, lifting motion, moving up and down the back two to three times.

13 Use a fanning technique: first, position yourself at the person's head area and place your thumbs at the top of the back, just below the neck and on either side of the spine. Use a fanning motion with your thumbs extended. Glide down towards the lower back. Do not apply pressure on the spine.

14 Next, move to the person's side. Apply twists by reaching around the far hip with one hand whilst resting the other hand on the near hip. With a fluid motion, pull one hand towards you as the other hand pushes away. Move up the back to the shoulder area, then come back down again. Repeat three times.

15 Finish with a couple of effleurage strokes on the back.

STUDENT TIP

There are many inexpensive handheld massage devices on the market, both electronic and static. You can even use a tennis ball.

EXERCISE 1.10 Three Self-Massage Techniques

Massage for headache
This massage is good for a throbbing headache.

1. Place your thumbs high on your cheekbones, by your ears.
2. Gently apply pressure to your temples in a circular motion with your fingertips.
3. Continue making circles as you move along your hairline until your fingertips meet in the middle of your forehead.

Neck massage
This massage will help to relieve tension and ease the pain.

1. Place two or three fingertips on the back of your neck where your neck meets your shoulders.
2. Apply firm pressure, and hold the area.
3. Release when the muscles feel more relaxed.
4. Roll your shoulders forward and backward slowly.
5. Repeat three times.

Massage for aching feet
This massage can help relieve aching feet after you have been on them all shift.

1. Sit in a comfortable chair with your feet bare.
2. Position a tennis ball under your feet.
3. Roll back and forth from the heel to the toe using firm pressure.
4. If you come across a painful or tender area, work the knot by rolling in small circles.
5. Do this exercise on both feet.
6. To add more pressure, try performing this technique whilst standing.

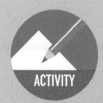

Chapter 1 Activity

Have a Luxurious Soak in the Bath

Place a few scented candles around the bathroom, and soak in a luxurious bubble bath.

If you don't have a bath, only a shower, you can purchase some essential oil steamers: you place these on the shower tray, furthest from the water, and the steam from the shower releases the essential oils from the steamer, scenting the bathroom like a spa.

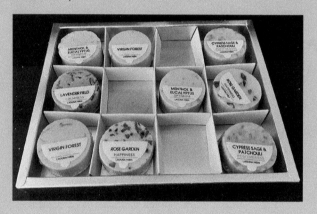

KEY POINTS

- NMC: Future Nurse: Standards of Proficiency for Registered Nurses (2018)
- Self-care
- Wellbeing
- Compassion fatigue
- Burnout
- Stress-relieving strategies

- Post-traumatic stress disorder
- Taking control
- Relaxation techniques
- Treating anxiety and psychological disorders – a new brain approach
- Eastern approaches for stress relief
- Acupuncture and acupressure
- Yoga
- Body massage
- Self-massage techniques
- Qigong
- Tai Chi

WEB RESOURCES

'NHS Lost One in Nine Staff in Pandemic': https://www.pressreader.com/uk/sunday-mirror/20220424/281582359187651

'NHS Sickness Absence During Covid-19 Pandemic': https://www.bmj.com/content/372/bmj.n471

Treating anxiety and psychological disorders by targeting new areas of the brain: http://www.mirror.co.uk/lifestyle/health/hope-scientists-targeting-new-area-26970056

Self-massage techniques: https://backintelligence.com/self-massage-techniques

Yoga: https://www.healthline.com/nutrition/13-benefits-of-yoga; www.yogainspires.co.uk

Yoga breathing: http://www.yogalondon.co.uk/blog/yoga-breathing-exercise

Burnout Syndrome: www.thoracic.org

NHS Employers (2018) Workforce Health and Wellbeing: www.nhsemployers.org?-?media/Employers/Publications?Health-and-wellbeing/NHS-Workforce-HWB-Framework

NHS Live Well: https://www.nhs.uk/live-well

Sleepio (a sleep-improvement program): https://good-thinking.uk/sleepio

Flamingo balance test: https://nypost.com/2022/06/22/flamingo-test-reveals-likelihood-of-dying-within-7-years

Taking control to combat stress: https://www.nhs.uk/mental-health/self-help/guides-tools-and-activities/tips-to-reduce-stress

Chapter 2

STRESS

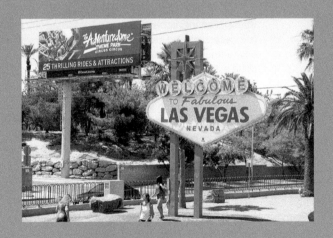

Wellbeing Strategies for Nurses, First Edition. Claire Boyd.
© 2023 John Wiley & Sons Ltd. Published 2023 by John Wiley & Sons Ltd.

LEARNING OUTCOMES

By the end of this chapter, you should have an understanding of the stress response, how to identify and manage stress, and how relaxation and complementary therapies can aid in stress relief. You will also have an overview of worldwide stress-relief strategies.

You don't necessarily have to book a fancy holiday somewhere like Las Vegas to relax and relieve your stressful life. In fact, the travel to and back from a holiday destination, with cancelled flights and lost luggage, may be extremely stressful in itself! Not to mention the empty bank balance on your return. So, what is stress?

WHAT IS STRESS?

Stress is an inevitable part of our lives, affecting everyone: it is a necessary and essential result of our interaction with our environment, enabling us to survive. For example, we need to be extra vigilant and alert when crossing a busy road or dealing with a violent patient.

This is known as the **stress response** or, more commonly, **fight or flight**. Our bodies are flooded with adrenaline, noradrenaline, and cortisol (hormones), prompting a number of alert responses, including faster heart rate and heightened muscle tension that allow us to respond quickly to the 'danger' (stressor) present.

Most people refer to stress in the negative, when the demands of life outweigh the ability of the individual to cope. Individuals undergoing stressful life events, such as bereavement, marital breakdown, work burnout, or depression may meet these criteria.

However, the **Yorkers-Dodson Law** states that a certain level of stress stimulation improves performance. An example is when athletes psych themselves up before races and perform to their best ability: you may have observed them slapping their thighs and jumping up and down, etc.

The majority of the stressors we encounter in life, we can deal with efficiently – indeed, they may even have a positive impact on our lives by providing excitement, interest, and challenge. Equally, too little stress can cause feelings of listlessness and under-stimulation, resulting in slow and inefficient performance and even depression. In short, stress is not all bad.

THE GENERAL ADAPTATION SYNDROME

In today's society, we may be unable to initiate the fight-or-flight response and thus have to carry on in a heightened state of stress Known as the **General Adaptation Syndrome**. When stressor is piled upon stressor, our bodies cannot restore balance (homeostasis) between encounters, and a high stress level is said to have incurred, which may become health-threatening. An example is when the body continues to manufacture stress chemicals over a prolonged period, and the immune system becomes depressed and poorly functioning.

The effects of high stress levels on the body, behaviour, thoughts, emotions, and health can be seen in Appendix A.

THE COST OF STRESS

It is estimated that workers take 13.4 million days off each year in the UK due to stress at work, at a cost of £3.8 billion. From a personal point of view, nursing can be considered a profession most affected by stress in the workplace due to chronic staff shortages, the constant culture of change, and violence at work – and this is before adding Covid and winter pressures to the equation!

DUTY OF CARE

Employers are duty-bound to protect the health of employees under the provision of the 1974 Health and Safety at Work Act. With nurses now taking civil actions in the courts in ever-increasing numbers, the government has recognised that stress is an important issue in the modern National Health Service and initiated the Commission for Health Improvement (CHI) to assess stress levels of healthcare workers; this now affects hospital star-rating status.

A MODEL OF STRESS?

A model of stress may be described as a set of scales (Figure 2.1a). When there is a prolonged imbalance between stressors and the ability to cope with chronic exhaustion, ill health is likely to occur (Figure 2.1b). Most healthcare staff I deliver my relaxation sessions to inform me that Figure 2.1b should have 'more stress loads' added to the scales for accuracy!

The heavier and more prolonged the load of stress and the less an individual's coping mechanisms, the more serious the symptoms of illness are likely to be. The key to a balanced (or homeostatic) stress life is to have effective coping strategies – the purpose of this book! As individuals, we all cope differently in different situations and have variable life experiences affecting our coping abilities. Figure 2.2 shows some of these variables.

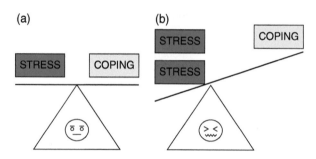

Figure 2.1 (a, b) A model of stress.

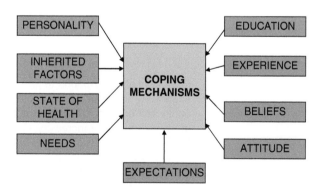

Figure 2.2 Coping mechanisms.

HOW DO WE KNOW WE ARE STRESSED?

The NHS suggest that we may be experiencing stress or burnout if we:

- Feel overwhelmed
- Have racing thoughts or difficulty concentrating
- Are irritable
- Feel constantly worried, anxious, or scared
- Feel a lack of self-confidence
- Have trouble sleeping or feel tired all the time (not related to long Covid, etc.)
- Avoid things or people we are having problems with
- Eat more or less than usual
- Drink or smoke more than usual

WHAT ARE THE CAUSES OF STRESS?

The NHS also suggests that some possible causes of stress may be:

- Our individual genes, upbringing, and life experiences
- Difficulties in our personal lives and relationships
- Big or unexpected life changes: e.g. moving house, having a baby or starting to care for someone (outside of work), death in the family, or losing a job
- Money difficulties, like debt or struggling to afford daily essentials
- Health issues, either for us or someone close to us
- Pregnancy and children
- Problems with housing, like conditions, maintenance, or tenancy
- A difficult or troubled work environment
- Feeling lonely and unsupported

STRESS-RESISTANT PERSONALITIES

It has been suggested that there is a **stress-resistant personality**: people with high levels of stress but low levels of illness. These people have been found to share three characteristics known as the three Cs:

- **Control** – A sense of purpose and direction in their life
- **Commitment** – To work, hobbies, social life, and family
- **Challenge** – Seeing changes in life as normal and positive rather than a threat

However, not everyone is born with these characteristics. Most of us have to learn effective strategies to cope with the influx of stressors: e.g. how to relax and let the stress wash over us. It should be noted that I have met some chilled people in my life, but never anyone said to be stress-resistant.

TYPE A AND TYPE B PERSONALITIES

Just as there is a stress-resistant personality, those studying the life sciences have also come across the character traits known as Type A and Type B personalities, developed by the cardiologists Fried and Rosenman. Their findings sought to explain why Type A personalities experience more coronary heart disease (CHD) and hypertension than Type B personalities.

DID YOU KNOW?

This research has been somewhat debunked today, as the initial study did not include females or take into account variables such as smoking and other lifestyle choices.

The study found that Type A personalities automatically trigger their stress responses when there is no real threat or challenge present; this personality type also tends to have an insufficient outlet for their constant sense of anger in response to trivial happenings, contributing to their adverse wellbeing. Figure 2.3 shows the personality traits.

A Type A personality is now referred to as a set of behavioural responses collectively known as the Type A behaviour pattern. There is also a perceived Type C behaviour pattern in individuals with the following traits:

- People pleasers
- Passive
- Patient
- Have difficulty expressing emotions like anger
- Suppress their own wants and needs

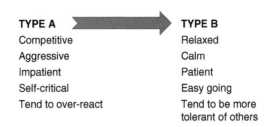

Figure 2.3 Personality traits.

It should also be recognised that humans are complex creatures and often do not fit into such regimental groups.

DID YOU KNOW?

If it's true that stress brings on weight loss, why am I not invisible?

DEALING WITH STRESS AND BURNOUT

The NHS have produced six top tips for dealing with stress and burnout, which can be viewed in Figure 2.4.

Split up the big tasks	If a task seems overwhelming and difficult to start, try breaking it down into small chunks. Then give yourself some credit for completing them.
Allow yourself some positivity	Take time to think about the good things in your life. Each day consider what went well and try to list three things that you are thankful for.
Challenge your thoughts	The way we think affects the way we feel. Try reframing your thoughts (which we will look at in Chapter 2).
Be more active	Being active can help burn off nervous energy. It will not make the stress disappear, but it can make it less intense.
Talk to someone	When we are struggling, talking to trusted friends, colleagues, or family or contacting a helpline can help.
Plan ahead	Planning out any tasks or events on a to-do list can really help with the stress levels.

Figure 2.4 Tips for dealing with stress and burnout.

Problem-Focused-Coping Stress Relief

Most stress relievers focus on changing your emotions. However, you may not get the stress relief you crave unless you change your actual environment: this is known as problem-focused coping, as opposed to emotion-focused coping. Problem-focused coping involves taking steps to remove the stressor from your life, as opposed to changing how you feel about the stressor.

Modern Technology

Smartphones, computers, and tablets are unavoidable parts of many people's everyday life, but using them too often may increase stress levels. A number of studies have linked excessive smartphone use and 'iPhone addiction' with increased stress levels and mental health disorders, and too much screen time may negatively affect sleep patterns.

EXERCISE 2.1   Reducing Screen Time

Reduce the time you spend on your electronic devices by an hour on day one. Then try to increase this to two hours on day two, and keep going until you reach a reduced but comfortable amount of screen time.

Stress Diaries

Keeping a stress diary is a good way to find your stress triggers. Then you can regain control by actively doing something about then.

EXERCISE 2.2   Keeping a Stress Diary

Buy a cheap notepad, and keep a stress diary. Write in your diary every day, and look for any emerging patterns that trigger your stress. Keeping this stress diary will help you identify changes you can make to your life.

After about a week, when you feel relaxed, look back at your diary and find where you can and will make these changes. If your stress comes from work, talk to your manager, colleagues, Occupational Health, etc.

CAN PLANNING HELP?

Dealing with stress effectively involves balancing the scales of coping and stressors (as previously discussed). This can be achieved by **reducing** demands by initiating any of the following:

- Learning to say 'No'
- Organising your life
- Being realistic about what you can achieve
- Delegating
- Seeking help when needed
- Prioritising

and by **increasing** demands by initiating any of the following:

- Taking up hobbies
- Joining evening classes
- Reappraising your job/role
- Learning relaxation/stimulation techniques
- Talking to friends/colleagues

Therefore, planning your tactics by changing your lifestyle may assist in reducing the adverse effects of stress on the body.

SETTING GOALS

Setting short, attainable goals can help us make life changes if stress is becoming overwhelming.

EXERCISE 2.3   Setting Goals

Write down what you would like to achieve in your life within a year. Find goals for categories of family, health, relationships, personal and leisure. Devise five steps for each category to help you achieve your goals. Visualise yourself achieving your goals, which will increase your motivation. When you achieve a goal, give yourself a reward. If you cannot reach a goal, don't feel disappointed; just modify your goal to achieve it.

HOW CAN RELAXATION THERAPIES HELP WITH STRESS?

Research has shown that relaxation training increases natural killer-cell activity within the body, thus strengthening the immune system. Natural killer cells attack harmful body invaders. Doctors often use relaxation methods such as meditation to treat patients with high blood and cholesterol levels.

There are a number of ways an individual experiencing high stress levels may bring about a state of relaxation, which we looked at in Chapter 1. There are also many other alternative therapies, such as Bach flower therapy, crystal therapy, homoeopathy, and using the power of the pyramids, to name just a few! However, this book will only look at the therapies I use and have been trained in as strategies to relieve stress and for which the research evidence is more robust.

EXERCISE 2.4   Humming

Humming to yourself helps to calm breathing and create vibrations that massage the section of the vagus nerve near your vocal cords. By activating this nerve, you actually turn off your fight-or-flight reflex, telling your brain and heart to calm down while triggering the release of feel-good neurotransmitters such as oxytocin to promote feelings of relaxation. Think of a tune, and have a hum when feeling stressed.

COMPLEMENTARY THERAPIES

So far, we have learned that the pressures and strains of everyday twenty-first century living and work have increased stress levels to all-time highs. Three-quarters of face-to-face or virtual consultations with general practitioners are due to stress-related complaints. Most GPs do not have time to talk through stress-related disorders to get to the root of the problem. It would seem that GPs are becoming more receptive to complementary therapies as treatments, recognising the holistic aspect of healthcare.

Holistic care targets the whole person – mind, body, and soul, rather than just the specific complaint as in the scientific (or medical) model of healthcare. Individuals are becoming disillusioned with certain aspects of conventional medicine. Many forms of anxiety and depression are treated with pills, which may be helpful in the short term but do not solve the underlying problems. In addition, side effects from taking conventional medicines have left many individuals feeling let down by the medical profession.

COMPLEMENTARY THERAPY SELF-CARE

Individuals may turn to excessive drinking, smoking, and/or drug abuse to cope with stress. However, many seek guidance to heal themselves. This has led to approximately 4–5 million people each year in the UK consulting a complementary practitioner. A **complementary therapy** is defined as a healthcare practice not currently an integral part of conventional medicine; such therapies encompass a diverse collection of ancient and modern beliefs. In the United States, an estimated $15 billion annually is spent on complementary and alternative medicine (CAM), with approximately one in four of the population using some aspect of complementary therapy. The reasons for using CAM are varied, but 'relaxation for stress' is deemed the number-one reason for visiting a CAM practitioner.

It has been suggested that ever-increasing numbers of individuals may be undertaking complementary therapy in part because people compare complementary therapies with nature – a more natural approach to health and illness.

Today, 65% of British doctors think that complementary medicine – such as massage, aromatherapy, and mindfulness – has a place in mainstream medicine. More nurses are also recognising the benefits of CAM, especially due to the often unbearable pressures they have had to endure during the coronavirus pandemic.

Members of the general public are recognising that high stress levels are detrimental to health and are choosing treatments to aid the relaxation process. Walk into any bookshop in the high street, and you can see an array of self-help books (admittedly, some make outlandish claims and are not evidence-based).

Massage Therapy

There is nothing nicer than a relaxing massage by a professional practitioner, especially using essential oils. We looked at massage therapy in Chapter 1 and will look at aromatherapy in Chapter 9. A simple, quick fix for stress is a simple self-administered hand massage. Exercise 2.4 shows how to perform this activity, which is a form of reflexology.

EXERCISE 2.5   Hand Massage

1   Place your thumb and index finger between the webbing of your opposite hand (you will first need to find the mound of muscle between the thumb and index finger), and massage firmly in a circular motion, pressing from above and beneath as close to the bone as you can get for three to five minutes.
2   Concentrate on your breathing, and release all your tension. Allow yourself to soak up the feelings of relaxation.
3   Now change hands, and repeat the process on the other hand.

Massaging your hands should help you redirect your mind towards relaxing in the moment. For an enhanced experience, essential oil massage blends or hand creams to rub in can be purchased from chemists or in health food shops.

TENSION

When stressed, we often carry tension in the neck and shoulder regions of our bodies. This can lead to aches and pains, headaches, and migraines. A good way to relieve this tension in the neck and shoulder is a self-massage, examples which can be seen in Exercise 2.6. Note that if you have any pain or injury in this area of the body, you should seek advice from your GP or physio before undertaking this exercise.

EXERCISE 2.6   Self-Massaging the Neck and Shoulders

1   **Relieving neck and shoulder tension:** Drop your shoulders down and back to relax them. Make a conscious effort to push your shoulders down and

away from your ears. This will help relax the trapezius muscles that connect your shoulders to your neck.

2 **Stretching the back of the neck:** Tuck your chin into your chest to stretch the back of your neck. Now stand up straight with your feet planted on the ground shoulder-width apart and your arms relaxed at your sides. Inhale deep into your diaphragm, and then lower your chin to your chest. Hold this position while you exhale for a slow count of 5. Return your head upright, and repeat this stretch 5–10 times per day or whenever you feel tense.

3 **Massaging the back muscles of the neck:** Put your left hand on the neck muscles behind your left ear. With a soft touch, use your fingers to apply gentle pressure to this area. Slowly turn your head to the right while applying the pressure. Make sure your fingers don't move and that it is just your head that is moving. Repeat this on the right side. Use your fingers to massage the same area of the neck with gentle circular movements to increase blood flow while releasing tension.

Note: Too much pressure can be unpleasant and even harmful, so keep the pressure as light as possible initially and gradually build up. Many years ago, when I was working towards my diploma in Indian head massage, I gave my poor daughter a migraine because I used too much pressure!

STRESS-RELIEF STRATEGIES FROM AROUND THE WORLD

Stress is universal. No one country has a monopoly, and no one country is stress-free. Countries worldwide have their own coping mechanisms. Figure 2.5 shows some of these countries' strategies. It should be noted that this does not mean that every individual residing in these countries practices these strategies. You can be a citizen in any country of the world to practice these strategies to enjoy their perceived benefit!

QUICK FIX FOR ANXIETY AND FEELINGS OF PANIC

According to Chinese theory, if you apply pressure to special points on the body, relief can be obtained from certain ailments. We have looked at this in chapter one. If you need a quick fix to relieve anxiety, tension or extreme pressure, why don't you try Exercise 2.7?

Country	Strategy
Russia	Many Russians enjoy 'Banya': a hot sauna. Individuals elsewhere can enjoy similar benefits by taking a hot shower. Research by Yale University states that pulsating water on the skin triggers brain and body responses boosting the mood naturally, due to the enveloping warmth mirroring emotional warmth.
Sweden	Many Swedes and Scandinavians enjoy 'Fika', which involves meeting with friends for coffee; this has been part of their culture since the 1700s. It is even better if accompanied by a sweet pastry or two! The Massachusetts Institute of Technology found that meeting and talking with friends can make us healthier.
Thailand	In Thailand, they enjoy a vigorous massage from a masseuse using their elbows and knees. The Touch Research Institute at the University of Miami shows that stimulating pressure receptors releases serotonin, the body's natural antidepressant. You can achieve some of the benefits of this by kneading the nape of your own neck and surrounding area of your body.
Argentina	People in Argentina often enjoy drinking 'mate', a hot herbal drink, especially in the presence of friends sitting in a circle passing the drink around to each other to sip – similar to the peace pipe. This is said to enable the individuals to feel connected amongst friends, much like they do in Sweden (and Belgium).
Belgium	As in Sweden and Argentina, sharing food and drink is a stress-relieving strategy, reiterating that you are a valued part of my network. The University of California states that this eating and drinking with friends releases a surge of calming oxytocin.
Ireland	The Irish often enjoy a brisk walk in the fresh winter air to energise and revive the brain. The University of Maryland School of Public Health Study found that exercise helps to reduce anxiety. Because there is less mood-boosting natural light during the winter months, it is especially helpful to get outside in the fresh air.
China	Women in China often do a warm foot soak called 'Zu Yu' before bed in order to relax. Adding Epsom salts (and two spoonfuls of baking soda) to the warm water foot bath has long been a strategy in many countries to relax and improve circulation.
India	In India they often have a good belly laugh before starting their day. Oxford University found that contracting stomach muscles trigger a surge of the calming feel-good endorphins, even after just a few minutes of laughter. Eating spicy food causes the body to produce the happy hormones.
Turkey	In Turkey they have 'keyif', which means to enjoy pleasurable things in the moment. This may mean listening to music, thereby distracting your brain and not thinking about anything stressful. Studies from Harvard University found that people subjected to freezing cold compresses were less likely to notice the discomfort when listening to music. This is about focusing on the positive and not the negative. This can also be replicated by writing down a list of the good things in your life and reading it when you next feel stressed and/or anxious.

Figure 2.5 Stress-relieving strategies from around the world.

Denmark	In Demark it gets dark very early in the afternoon, so they have created 'hygge' – cosy. This is about visiting each other's houses, not rushing, and being happy. We can all replicate this by entertaining our friends in our homes, making sure we do not get stressed if preparing food or cleaning the house! Nothing needs to be perfect – it is about having fun with your friends (who don't care that your carpet needs hoovering)!
United Kingdom	Nothing is quite as quintessential as making a 'cuppa' in times of stress in the UK. Research shows that black tea contains catechins and theobromine, chemicals that can help reduce the symptoms of anxiety and increase the amount of serotonin the body makes. Silymarin, a soluble antioxidant, is also thought to help with these symptoms of stress, with L-theanine being the most powerful. Green tea has exceptionally high levels of L-theanine. Peppermint tea contains menthol, a naturally occurring muscle relaxant. So the next time you feel stressed, do the British thing and put the kettle on!

Figure 2.5 (*Continued*)

EXERCISE 2.7 Acupressure for Anxiety and Feelings of Panic

Find the spot: one finger width below the crease inside your wrist. Press your thumb on the skin directly in line with your little finger.
Hold the pressure for around one minute or until you feel calm.

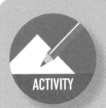

Chapter 2 Activity

ACTIVITY

Choose one of these six stress-relieving activities to do today – the choice is yours!

Peel and eat an orange. Researchers studying depression have found that citrus fragrances boost feelings of wellbeing and alleviate stress by increasing levels of norepinephrine found to affect our moods.

Tidy up. Studies show that having a mess around us can cause stress. So, have a bit of a declutter and donate anything you no longer use or need to charity, sell it on Gumtree, etc.

Eat some nuts. B vitamins, zinc, magnesium, and omega oils are quickly used up by the body when we are stressed, and nuts are a good source of these elements.

Exercise. Walk up the stairs instead of using the lift, or go for a short jog: Studies have shown that regular physical exercise can reduce stress levels.

Bake a cake. Studies show that repetitive tasks such as weighing, chopping, and mixing can be therapeutic due to their meditative nature.

Try cupping. If you are at work and feeling stressed, try 'cupping': rub your hands together vigorously for one minute. Then immediate cup them over your closed eyes for five seconds whilst you breathe deeply. The warmth and darkness are comforting, and resting your eyes can also help to relax your whole body. Note: If you wear glasses, it is a good idea to remove these first – D'oh!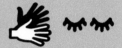

KEY POINTS

- What is stress?
- General Adaptation Syndrome
- The cost of stress
- Duty of care
- A model of stress
- How do we know if we are stressed?
- What are the causes of stress?
- Stress-resistant personalities
- Type A and Type B personalities
- Dealing with stress and burnout
- Can planning help?
- How can relaxation therapies help with stress?
- Complementary therapies
- Massage therapy
- Self neck massage
- Stress-relief strategies from around the world

WEB RESOURCES

- **NHS: Every Mind Matters:** https://www.nhs.uk/every-mind-matters//mental-health-issues/stress
- **Signs and symptoms of stress:** https://www.mind.org.uk/information-support/types-of-mental-health-problems/stress/signs-and-symptoms-of-stress/
- **Self-massage for neck pain:** https://uppercervicalawareness.com/neck-pain-relief-try-these-4-self-massage-techniques

Chapter 3
. . . .
SLEEP WELL

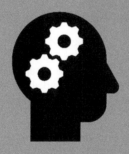

Wellbeing Strategies for Nurses, First Edition. Claire Boyd.
© 2023 John Wiley & Sons Ltd. Published 2023 by John Wiley & Sons Ltd.

LEARNING OUTCOMES

By the end of this chapter, you will have an understanding of the importance of a good night's sleep, techniques for getting a good night's sleep, and disturbances that prevent getting a good night's sleep, including orthosomnia, night-shift work, and shift work sleep disorder.

We all have times when our brains are still whirling at the end of a hectic shift and we find it difficult to shut down and relax. Perhaps this inability to wind down encroaches on our ability to sleep. Reaching for alcohol or sleeping pills as a quick fix is not the best option long-term.

SLEEPLESS NIGHTS

One in three of us suffers from poor sleep, which can be caused by numerous things such as stress, taking our work home with us, and financial worries, to name but three.

Lack of sleep does not just cause a lack of focus and/or being in a constant bad mood: regularly losing sleep can make us more prone to serious medical conditions, including heart disease and diabetes. Lack of sleep can also shorten our life expectancy; we can therefore say that a solid night's sleep is essential for a long and healthy life.

Most of us need around seven to eight hours of good-quality sleep at night to function properly, but some of us need more and some of us need less. Many of us who do not get the requisite hours of sleep may experience fatigue, a lack of focus, and a short temper.

DID YOU KNOW?

Scientists from Cambridge University (2022) have discovered that seven hours of sleep a night is best for healthy brain ageing. Longer or shorter periods can lead to anxiety, depression, and worse overall wellbeing. The study questioned 500 000 adults between ages 38 and 73 about their sleep patterns and asked them to perform various cognitive tests. Seven hours of sleep was found to be the ideal amount for the brain to rid itself of toxins and the optimum amount to boost mood, memory, and attention span.

An occasional night without sleep may make us tired and irritable the next day, but it should not harm our health. However, after several sleepless nights, the mental and physical effects become more serious. We now begin to find it more difficult to concentrate and make decisions. Our risk of injury and accidents also increases.

Continuous lack of sleep can affect our overall health and make us more prone to serious medical conditions, such as obesity, hypertension, heart disease, and diabetes.

Quality of Sleep Rather than Quantity

A study by Cambridge University and Fudan University in China found that it is better to have fewer hours of good sleep than it is to have seven or eight hours of broken sleep. Other researchers have come up with a formula that works out how well you sleep (and also offers solutions for those who do not sleep well). The formula is:

$$\text{Sleep quality} = \frac{(CT \times Bt) + c/Ha +}{S + L + (H \times D)}$$

A score of 2 is a great night's sleep, 1 is average, and 0 means you are tossing and turning all night.

KEY

T = Tiredness. Calculated by working out the number of hours since your last overnight sleep minus the number of hours spent napping plus the hours of physical exercise taken during the day.
Bt = Your bedtime that night divided by your their normal bedtime.
C = Comfort. Calculated as the comfort of a pillow, plus bedding, plus a mattress, minus 9. Scores for each item of bedding are worked out by rating them from 1 (very uncomfortable) to 5 (very comfortable).
Ha = Average hours awake. For most people, this will be about 16 hours.
S = Sounds, rated from 1 (very soft) to 5 (very loud, irregular, and disturbing).
L = Light, including any light in the room (illuminated clocks, etc.). It is rated from 0.1 (very soft light) to 2 (very bright blue spectrum light).
H = Heat. Calculated by working out the difference in degrees between the room temperature and 16–17 °C and dividing by 10.

D = Duvet appropriateness for the room temperature, rated from 0 (compensates perfectly for room temperature) to 3 (does not compensate well and leaves you far too hot or too cold).

Table 3.1 shows what the experts suggest for a good night's rest.

Table 3.1 Good sleep.

20 minutes of daylight	Exposure to daylight kickstarts our body's processes and gives us a natural feeling of sleepiness about 14 hours later. It is light and dark exposure that sets our circadian rhythm. It is important to expose ourselves to this amount of natural light at the start of the day – this could be by sitting next to a window whilst having breakfast or sitting out in the garden. For shift workers, a SAD lamp will have the same effect.
30 grams of fibre	Eating the right amount of fibre can improve sleep quality, increasing the time we spend in the deep-sleep stages, which is crucial to waking up feeling refreshed and rested. The NHS recommends eating 30 grams of fibre each day, starting with high-fibre breakfast cereals.
6 minutes of reading	A study from the University of Sussex showed that it could take just 6 minutes of reading at bedtime to lower your stress levels by 68% and significantly relax you.
18° room temperature	The optimum temperature for bedrooms is just 18 °C. Our bodies are programmed to decrease slightly in temperature in the evenings, so having a cool room is essential for good-quality sleep.
10 deep breaths	Taking yoga breaths before bed is said to balance your nervous system. The breath lowers the heart rate, dissolves tension in the body, and allows the brain to change from tension and stress mode to rest and sleep mode. Chapter 4 shows yoga breathing techniques.
10 minutes of calming sounds	Natural sounds such as rain, waves, and bird song can be soothing. This is because the sounds are at a certain pitch, and our brain perceives them as non threatening.
90 minutes before trying again	Sleep is like surfing, because we need to catch the wave: we may feel sleepy but want to finish what we are doing or watching on the television. By the time we have finished what we are doing, we have missed the wave and no longer feel sleepy. We then need to wait for the next wave, and it may take 60–90 minutes until we feel sleepy again. That way we are far more likely to go straight to sleep rather than lying awake and feeling frustrated.

Sleep Schedules

The NHS suggests that sleep problems usually sort themselves out within a month. Longer stretches of poor sleep can affect our lives, making usually manageable tasks harder due to extreme tiredness. If poor sleep becomes regular, it may be that you are experiencing insomnia. Insomnia can last for months or even years unless you do something about it, such as changing your sleeping habits: e.g. sticking to a sleep schedule, perhaps by setting aside no more than eight hours for sleep. Other techniques to help you fall asleep are the pre-bedtime preparations, which can be seen in Table 3.2.

Table 3.2 NHS's suggested pre-bedtime preparations.

Winding down	You may like to read as a means of winding down prior to sleep, or undertaking some light stretching or relaxation techniques. These should be performed an hour before putting head to pillow.
Temperature	The bedroom should be a comfortable temperature, ideally running a little cool. Bed attire should be comfortable.
No electronics	All electronics should be disconnected (i.e. laptops, phones, tablets, etc.) due to the blue light stimulating the brain and making it harder to fall asleep.
Lighting	Ideally the lights should be dimmed to help your eyes relax and get the brain prepared for sleep mode.
Food	Big meals should be avoided in the lead-up to sleep, as should spicy foods, caffeine, and alcohol.
Scent	Lavender essential oil has a relaxation effect, and pillow sprizer blends can be readily purchased to enhance the calming effect of the sleeping environment.

EXERCISE 3.1 Guided Visualisation for Sleep

When you experience difficulty sleeping, with your mind going 100 miles an hour, try this mini guided visualisation for sleep:

1   Turn off your electronic devices, including your phone. After taking a nice warm bath with a lovely scented bubblebath, get into your PJs and go to bed.
2   Turn off the lights, and settle down comfortably on your bed. Close your eyes.
3   Begin to focus on your breathing, taking nice deep breaths in and out. Feel the bed rising up to meet and support you, and allow yourself to grow heavier and heavier with each breath.
4   Feel your body sinking into the softness of your bed. As your body becomes still, your mind begins to drift.
5   In your mind, visualise a green meadow, soft, calm, and peaceful. You feel the breeze blowing against your cheek. You smell the pure, clean air. You feel the soft grass under your feet.
6   You listen, and you hear the stillness of nature. You breathe and look around the meadow. You see the valley and the mountains in the far distance. You fill your lungs with pure air – taking deep breaths in and out, in and out.
7   Your mind becomes clear as you focus on this scene. Tell yourself:
    •   I am calm and peaceful.
    •   I am calm and peaceful.
    •   I am calm and peaceful.
8   Allow yourself to drift off.

The Benefits of a Good Night's Sleep

According to the National Health Service, a good night's sleep can boost your health in the ways shown in Table 3.3.

Table 3.3 The benefits of a good night's sleep.

Sleep boosts immunity.	A prolonged lack of sleep can disrupt your immune system so you'll be less able to fend of bugs.
Sleep can help you stay slim.	Sleep-derived people have reduced levels of leptin (the chemical that makes us feel full) and increased levels of ghrelin (the hunger-stimulating hormone).

Table 3.3 (*Continued*)

Sleep boosts mental well-being.	Chronic sleep debt may lead to long-term mood disorders like clinical depression and generalised anxiety disorder in adults.
Sleep prevents diabetes.	Sleep debt may lead to type 2 diabetes by changing the way the body processes glucose (used by the body for energy).
Sleep increase sex drive.	Sleep debt may lead to a loss of libido (reduced sex drive) and less of an interest in sex. Men who experience sleep apnoea also tend to have lower testosterone levels, which can also lower libido.
Sleep wards off heart disease.	Longstanding sleep deprivation seems to be associated with increased heart rate, an increase in blood pressure, and higher levels of certain chemicals linked with inflammation, which may put extra strain on your heart.
Sleep increases fertility.	Difficulty conceiving a baby has been claimed as one of the effects of sleep deprivation in both men and women. Apparently, regular sleep disruption can affect fertility by reducing the secretion of reproduction hormones.

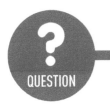

QUESTION

Question   Have you ever wondered why you feel tired after eating a big meal?

Answer Eating large portions of food, such as a Sunday roast, can overload your digestive system and make it work extra hard to digest all you have just eaten. Therefore, a lot of blood is diverted from the brain, and that makes you feel sleepy. This is the effect when we drink alcohol. Certain foods, such as turkey, cheese, and eggs, contain tryptophan, an essential amino acid; it helps our bodies produce the mood hormone serotonin, which helps us relax and makes us feel sleepy.

WORRYING ABOUT NOT GETTING ENOUGH SLEEP

Research tells us that women generally have more trouble drifting off to sleep than men (but it doesn't tell us why)! In the UK, 36% of all adults struggle to get to sleep at least once a week, with one in five having trouble every single night. Once we have difficulty sleeping, we may then get anxious about sleep, tossing and turning and worrying that we can't perform properly at work the next day. This worry is called **orthosomnia** – disrupted sleep caused by an obsession about getting a good night's sleep.

Orthosomnia Remedies

Many of us, after experiencing sleep deprivation and worrying about it, have tried remedies for a good night's sleep that we may have been told about by friends and colleagues. But are they supported by scientific evidence? We all know about how our ancestors used honey in wound care, and the research showed that this actually worked. What about these sleep hacks? Do they actually work? In Table 3.4, we look at six 'sleep tips' coupled with a review of the evidence.

Table 3.4 Tips for a good night's sleep.

Remedy for sleep	Verdict
Drink lettuce tea Put a few leaves into a mug of hot water and drink before bedtime.	Lettuce contains lactucin, so boiling down the lettuce and drinking the water could act as a natural sedative. However, you need to boil down quite a significant number of leaves to produce enough lactucin. Drinking warm water may have a calming placebo effect.
Massage your wrists. Massage each wrist in a circular motion for 30–60 seconds to reduce anxiety and improve sleep quality.	Massaging turns on the body's parasympathetic nervous system, responsible for reducing heart rate and lowering blood pressure, which could aid sleep.
Create a pillow wall. If you share a bed, place a wall of pillows between you and your partner.	If your partner snores or encroaches on your space in the bed, this physical barrier may muffle sounds and offer a little comfort so you don't get so 'wound up' each night.

Table 3.4 (*Continued*)

Remedy for sleep	Verdict
Eat kiwi fruit. Eating some kiwi fruit is said to increase the amount and quality of sleep.	According to a study, eating kiwi can improve sleep onset, duration, and efficiently in adults. This has been found to be particularly true for those with sleep disorders, due to the sleep-inducing chemical messenger serotonin.
Tape your mouth. Placing a small strip of porous medically approved tape over the centre of the mouth to ensure that you breathe out of your nose and not the mouth to reduce snoring.	If you sleep with your mouth open, the tongue falls back, blocking the airways and making the process of breathing harder. The use of porous medical tape improves snoring and obstructive sleep apnoea (OSA). With OSA, the airway is completely blocked for a few seconds until your brain wakes you up. OSA can lead to strokes and heart attacks.
Eat some chocolate. Eat some dark chocolate for a peaceful night's sleep.	Dark chocolate contains high levels of magnesium, which helps you to fall sleep quicker and for longer. Magnesium is also good for anxiety. The downside is that sugar has the opposite effect on peaceful sleep. Nuts and bananas are high in magnesium and contain less sugar.

EXERCISE 3.2   Military Sleep Technique

This breathing and muscle relaxation system was developed by the military to enable soldiers to fall asleep at any time and any place, even on the battlefield where pandemonium is all around! It has been suggested that using this technique enables sleep to occur within two minutes:

1   Start by relaxing your muscles in your forehead.
2   Relax your eyes, your cheeks, and your jaw. Focus on your breathing.
3   Now go down to your neck and your shoulders. Make sure your shoulders are not tensed up, and drop them as low as you can; keep your arms loose by your sides, including your hands and fingers. Imaging a warm sensation going from your head down to your fingertips before travelling from your heart to your toes.
4   Take a deep breath and slowly exhale, relaxing your chest, your stomach, down to your thighs, knees, legs, and feet.

5   Try to clear your mind of stress, and then imagine one of these two scenarios:
  • You are lying in a canoe on a calm lake with nothing but a clear blue sky above you.
  • You are lying in a black velvet hammock in a pitch black room.

If you feel as though you are getting distracted, repeat the words 'Don't think, don't think' for 10 seconds.

SLEEP DEPRIVATION

When we are sleep-deprived, apart from feeling over-tired, we may also feel sluggish, weak, and unproductive and make more mistakes. Table 3.5 shows 12 other signs of sleep deprivation and how they affect us.

Table 3.5 12 signs of sleep deprivation.

Always being hungry	When we are not well rested, the production of ghrelin can increase. This hormone is often known as the 'hunger hormone'. Therefore, when the brain does not get enough energy from sleep, it may try to get energy from foods – often fatty and sugary ones. A 2008 study in the *Journal of Sleep Research* found that after just one night of sleep deprivation, ghrelin levels acutely increased. Another hormone affected by sleep deprivation is the satiety hormone, leptin, which is responsible for telling us when we are repleat and to stop eating.
Gaining weight	With an increased appetite, it is no wonder another symptom of sleep deprivation is weight gain. A lack of sleep can have a direct affect on our metabolism, slowing it down. A study in the *Annals of Internal Medicine* (2012) found that just 4-1/2 hours of sleep for four days straight reduce the ability of fat cells to respond to insulin (a hormone responsible for regulating energy) by 30%.
Being more impulsive	Sleep deprivation enhances our impulsivity to negative stimuli, meaning we may react before we have actually processed all the information concerning a situation. A study in 2007 in the *Journal of Physiology and Behavior* found that patients with impulse control disorders often reported sleep disorders; and in healthy individuals, a lack of sleep impaired their cognitive decision-making and changed the way they weighed risk. Risk-taking as a behaviour decreased in women but remained the same in sleep-deprived men.

Table 3.5 (*Continued*)

Memory problems	Sleep deprivation has a negative impact on memory function, due to lack of protein synthesis in the hippocampus section of the brain, which controls memory, learning, and emotions. A report in the *Journal of Behavioural Brain Research* (2012) found that sleep deprivation induces oxidative stress (an imbalance between free radicals and antioxidants in the body), which further impairs learning and memory processes. Vitamin E, which is a strong antioxidant, counteracts the negative impact of sleep deprivation on memory function (known as chronic sleep deprivation-induced cognitive impairment). However, vitamin E is not a quick-fix, as if you want to strengthen your memory, you still need adequate sleep.
Having trouble making decisions	Sleep deprivation can affect sleep and higher-level cognitive processing, such as problem-solving or time-management abilities, making these tasks even more difficult to achieve. A study in the journal *Sleep* (2009) found that poor sleep hinders our ability to react quickly and make the right decisions.
Motor skills problems	A 2014 study published by the National Institutes of Health suggested that sleep deprivation negatively impacts motor and reverses learning and memory, meaning when we are tired, there's a lapse in how we function neurologically. With lowered reaction time and concentration comes more difficulty with movement because we can't process particularly well, meaning we may experience more trips and falls, etc.
Fluctuating emotions	When we are sleep deprived, we may become more over-reactive to emotional stimuli. A study in the *Journal of Sleep Medicine* (2008) showed that a lack of proper sleep makes us not only more emotional but also less emotionally intelligent. It also lessens our constructive thinking skills, meaning we are less able to express control or even be aware of our emotions.
Becoming poorly more often	A study in the *Archives of Internal Medicine* (2009) found that individuals who got less than seven hours of sleep were nearly three times as likely to develop a cold than those who get eight hours or more of rest at night. The immune system produces cytokines whist we sleep, which are proteins that help protect against infections and inflammation; so, a few nights of poor sleep could lower the body's defences against viruses.

(*Continued*)

Table 3.5 (*Continued*)

Sight problems	When we are fatigued, we are unable to control the muscles of the eyes as well, due to the ciliary muscle tiring (which controls the focusing of the eyes). A study in 1999 showed a strong correlation between children who slept with their light on and near-sightedness later in life. For adults, the modern blue light of technology, such as televisions, iPods, laptops, phones, etc., can contribute to poor sleep.
Skin problems	Our skin can often be a good indicator of our general health. An *American Journal of Clinical Dermatology* study in 2014 found that poor sleepers had higher levels of transdermal water loss than those experiencing good sleep, therefore ageing their skin prematurely. Good sleepers had 30% greater skin barrier recovery, with poor sleepers generally looking more fatigued, often with dark circles under the eyes, saggy eyelids, fine lines and wrinkles, drooping corners of the mouth, paler skin, and more likelihood of experiencing acne. This is due to disruption of the circadian rhythm, causing abrupt biological changes and imbalances in the skin. Sleep deprivation can also make us reach for the caffeine for a quick fix, which contributes to occasional acne, as can cigarettes. During sleep, the skin restores itself by producing collagen, with the cells regenerating; DNA repair is also boosted during sleep.
Micro-sleeps	When we are sleep-deprived, the brain can actually force the body to sleep for a few seconds, whether we like it or not! These are called micro-sleeps, and they can be extremely dangerous if operating machinery or even driving. The National Highway Traffic Safety Administration estimated that in 2009, 2.2–2.6% of total fatal crashes involved drowsy driving.
Growth problems	The human growth hormone (HGH) is released when we are asleep. This is why babies undergo rapid growth and need to sleep so much. The *Nursing Management Journal* suggests that children aged between 5 and 10 years need to sleep for 10–11 hours, and children between 10 and 17 years require about 8–9 hours. A study in the *Journal of Clinical Endocrinology and Metabolism* suggested that a lack of sleep leaves us with fewer hormones, thus stifling growth and development.

Source: https://www.health.com/mind-body/signs-of-sleep-deprivation.

Food and Sleep Deprivation

There are foods that you should avoid for better sleep and foods that help you get a better night's sleep. First and foremost, you should avoid eating less than three hours before bedtime, as you will still be digesting the food instead of using the bloodflow and energy to repair your mind and body.

Foods to avoid for a better night's sleep: Processed foods and foods high in calories, sugar, and fat. These are known as **high glycaemic index** (GI) foods and are typically broken down quickly by the body, which causes a rapid spike in blood sugar followed by a sudden crash later.

Foods to help you get better sleep: To regulate the blood sugar, you need to include a lot of low-GI foods and medium-GI foods in your diet (see Table 3.6). These foods are broken down more slowly by the body and cause a gradual rise in blood sugar levels over time. Medium-GI foods include orange juice, honey, basmati rice, and wholemeal and high-grain bread. Low-GI foods include unprocessed fish and meat, eggs, soy products, beans, fruit, milk, pasta, oats, and lentils.

Table 3.6 Six foods that can help you get a good night's sleep.

Fish	• **High in vitamin B6** • **Encourages the production of the sleep hormone melatonin** • **Good source of vitamin D and omega-3 fatty acids, which are important in the production of serotonin (the happiness hormone) known to aid sleep**
Bananas	• **High in vitamin B6** • **Contains magnesium (linked to lower stress levels), potassium (acts as a muscle-relaxant), and melatonin (encourages better sleep)**
Almonds	• **Good source of low-fat protein** • **Contains magnesium and tryptophan (an amino acid that plays a crucial role in the production of serotonin and large amounts of melatonin)**

(Continued)

Table 3.6 (*Continued*)

Milk, dairy, and soy milk	• Contains tryptophan • Calcium helps the tryptophan to manufacture melatonin, which has a sleep-inducing effect.
Sour cherry juice	• Certain varieties of sour cherries (not sweet cherries) such as, Richmond, English Morello, and Montmorency contain above-average concentrations of melatonin, which as we know encourages sleep
Chamomile tea	• Contains apigenin, a chemical compound that binds to specific receptors in the brain that help to decrease anxiety and initiate sleep

The Paradoxical Sleep Technique

The effects of sleep deprivation on our health have been well studied, including the damage it can do to our brains, which can increase the odds of us experiencing dementia and Alzheimers. One branch of insomnia research suggests using 'paradoxical intention' for restorative slumber. This method involves persuading ourselves to challenge and engage with a feared behaviour: in this case, the fear of not being able to sleep.

TERMINOLOGY

Paradoxical: Seemingly absurd or self-contradictory. Example: If I tell you **not** to think of an elephant, the first picture you conjure up in your mind will probably be an elephant.

Paradoxical Intention works by telling yourself that you are not going to sleep – that you are going to stay awake at all costs. You just lie in bed with your eyes wide open, forcing yourself to stay awake. After some time, you will feel tired and fall asleep.

Sleep scientists suggest that in paradoxical intention, you are actually setting out to do the thing you are trying to avoid, thereby breaking the fear cycle. By undertaking the feared or disliked behaviour, you eventually reduce the anxiety around it. You are, in effect, prescribing the symptom you want to avoid, meaning the performance anxiety related to sleep is reduced.

The paradoxical intention sleeping hack works best when combined with other sleep therapy strategies as seen in Table 3.1, although it can be effective on its own.

CLEAN SLEEPING

This is a wellness trend popularised by Gwyneth Paltrow and is about restoring good sleeping patterns and setting the body on a natural path to getting a good night's rest, starting by winding yourself down before bedtime. We have already looked at some of the principles of getting a good night's sleep, but the principle of clean sleeping utilises many of them – in short, they are nothing new.

Clean sleeping includes:

- Getting at least seven to nine hours of sleep every night
- Maintaining a consistent sleep schedule (and aiming to be in bed by 10 p.m. each night): i.e. going to bed and waking up at the same time each day, seven days a week.
- Avoiding technology before bed (because blue light suppresses sleep-inducing melatonin). Leave your phone outside the bedroom, and buy an old fashioned alarm clock instead. Also turn off the television at least an hour before bedtime.
- Limiting caffeine after 2 p.m. each day.
- Having a 12-hour fasting window each day and avoiding eating at least two hours before bedtime.
- Writing down your thoughts and concerns if you feel anxious before going to bed.

You can also include in your clean sleeping practice the meditative practice of yoga nidra. This involves preparing for clean sleeping by lying back in a comfortable position, closing your eyes, and then continuing as follows:

- The first goal of the preparation is to reunite with your body – you can do this by undertaking a body scan (see Chapter 13).

- The second goal of the preparation is to reunite with your mind – you can do this by acknowledging your thoughts and emotions and then letting them pass.
- The third goal of the preparation is to be mindful of the present moment – you can do this by focusing on your breathing, such as using the box breathing technique (see Chapter 13).

Next begins the yoga nidra meditation, such as the Water Lily script.

EXERCISE 3.3   Water Lily Script

You are lying on your back on a large water lily, floating on top of a vast motionless ocean in a faraway land. The water is completely still, and you feel completely safe and at peace. The air is warm as you feel the steady heat of the sun beat down upon your face and body, cleansing you.

You are happy and comfortable, drifting on your back with your eyes closed, safe, encased all around by your strong, thick water lily, miles from anything but calm open water.

The strength of the water lily makes you feel protected and safe. It is thick, and the water cannot even think about seeping in.

Rest here, drifting happily, without a care in the world.

As you drift, content, warm, safe, and protected, your awareness begins to fade away, and you drift off to sleep.

WORKING NIGHT SHIFTS

You don't need to be a rocket scientist to know that shift work can be harmful to sleep. As humans, our body clocks are designed for us to be active in the day and asleep at night, so our natural circadian rhythm is disrupted when we do otherwise. Research into working night shifts tell us working these antisocial hours are linked to prematurely ageing the brain, dulling our intellectual ability, and breast cancer. Working night shifts is also linked to obesity, as employees who have to sleep during the day burn fewer calories than when sleeping at night.

Nurses are not the only employees who work shifts, but in common perhaps is the inability to achieve a good sleep. Some shift workers may work permanent night shifts, a week of night shifts, or mixed rotating shifts, making it extremely difficult to get into any kind of routine. Without an effective routine, we may have difficulty achieving daytime sleep, resulting in issues such as drowsiness, fatigue in the workplace due to poor concentration, absenteeism, accidents, errors, injuries, etc.

Shift Work Sleep Disorder

An estimated 20% of the population in industrialised countries work in a job with nonstandard shifts. Approximately 10–38% of these workers suffer from shift work disorder (also known as shift work sleep disorder – SWSD), which is categorised as a circadian rhythm sleep disorder.

DID YOU KNOW?

Shift work sleep disorder is a condition marked by excessive sleepiness when awake or an inability to sleep when needed.

A circadian rhythm sleep disorder is when there is a misalignment between the body and the circadian rhythms that regulate the sleep–wake cycle. Other circadian rhythm sleep disorders include delayed and advanced sleep–wake phase disorder, irregular sleep–wake rhythm disorder, and our old favourite, jet lag.

Circadian rhythms are largely guided by natural light and darkness. During the day, the retinas in our eyes perceive sunlight, and signals are sent to the brain to release hormones like cortisol that help us feel alert and energised. As the light fades when the sun sets, the brain produces another hormone, melatonin, that induces feelings of sleepiness and relaxation.

SWSD specifically relates to circadian misalignment related to a work schedule that overlaps with a traditional sleep–wake cycle. Excessive sleepiness (insomnia) whilst awake and recurring sleep loss are the defining symptoms of shirt work disorder. To have a diagnoses of SWSD, individuals must have symptoms that occur for at least one month despite attempts to get enough sleep each day.

Complications of Shift Work Sleep Disorder

It is vital to find remedies for SWSD, as if it is left untreated, it can cause serious complications such as those in Table 3.7.

Table 3.7 Complications of shift work sleep disorder.

Mood problems	Individuals experiencing **SWSD** may avoid interacting with their co-workers and may also feel less inclined to socially engage with friends and family members when not at work. SWSD can also cause people to feel impatient, irritable, and unable to cope with problems or conflicts. People with SWSD are at a higher risk of depression compared to those who do not have the disorder.
Poor work performance	Individuals with SWSD often struggle to concentrate, remember things, and pay attention – not ideal in the nursing profession. This can also translate into reduced performance at work, with possible added costs for employers.
Added health problems	SWSD and general sleep loss can worsen any underlying health problems, including gastrointestinal, metabolic, reproduction, and cardiovascular issues. A good night's sleep is needed to restore the body and maintain good immune health. Shift work has also been linked to breast cancer incidences.
Low testosterone	In some individuals, shift work can affect their testosterone levels, which often presents in fatigue, low energy, and low libido.
Substance abuse	Many individuals, experiencing sleep disorders tend to self-medicate with drugs and/or alcohol. This can lead to substance abuse or dependency if the sleep disorder persists.
Higher accident risk	SWSD decreases alertness and reaction time, putting workers at higher risk of making errors or being involved in accidents. These individuals are also at higher risk of getting into a road traffic incident on their way to and from their workplace due to their drowsiness.

Shift Work Sleep Disorder Treatments

Successfully adapting to shift work requires coaching the body to sleep at times that may feel unnatural. Many shift workers find that they can minimise the symptoms of SWSD using a combination of medication, bright light therapy, and lifestyle modification.

Medication

Melatonin supplements	Melatonin is a sleep-promoting hormone usually produced in the evening after sundown. Taking melatonin supplements at other times of the day may help your body prepare for sleep.
Wakefulness-promoting medication	Two medications that may be administered to treat SWSD are modafinil and armodafinil. Taken one hour before work, these drugs may help to boost alertness.
Sleep-promoting medication	Prescription sleep aids such as benzodiazepines can be used to help facilitate sleep for shift workers, but they may be habit forming.

Note: Before taking any non-prescribed medication, you should first discuss it with your doctor.

Bright Light Therapy

Light therapy and light avoidance	Exposure to bright light can keep you awake and delay when you start to feel sleepy before your shift. After the shift, in the middle of the day, wearing dark sunglasses when you leave work may help to minimise the sunlight's alertness-promoting effects. Light can affect your sleep even when your eyes are closed, so it is a good idea to use blackout curtains/blinds and eye masks to sleep.

Lifestyle Modifications

Minimise disturbances.	Turn off phones. Ask household members to be quiet when you are sleeping, as best as they can. Use blackout curtains/blinds, eye masks, and ear plugs.
Catch up on sleep.	Many shift workers accumulate sleep debt. This lost sleep may be partially recovered on days off.
Take naps.	Very short naps during your work shift may boost alertness, as long as they fit in with your current sleep–wake schedule. Limiting these naps to 20 minutes can help to avoid the grogginess that occurs when waking up from a deep sleep.
Stay alert.	Many shift workers find that caffeine or other stimulants helps them stay alert on the job, but caffeine should not be consumed too close to the sleep period as it may impair sleep.
Stay active.	Carefully timed exercise may help regulate the sleep–wake cycle for shift workers.
Eat a balanced diet.	To avoid blood sugar spikes and fluctuations in energy, try to eat a diet rich in fruit and vegetables and low in high-sugar or processed foods.
Practice clean sleep.	Keep a regular bedtime routine, using relaxation techniques and avoiding blue light before bed.

DID YOU KNOW?

During heatwaves, the hot weather can affect our sleep cycles. But did you know you can reduce the heat in your bedroom by 20–30% using a roll of aluminium foil and a spray bottle of soapy water? Spray the soapy water on the windows and then put the foil on them, with the shiny side facing outward. The foil acts as a huge sun reflector.

BREATHING YOURSELF TO SLEEP

As with most relaxation techniques, the process often starts with deep breathing. The next exercise is said to aid the sleep process.

EXERCISE 3.4   5-5-5-5 Breathing Technique

This exercise is said to help you drift off to sleep and help you sleep more deeply:

1   Breathe in for five seconds.
2   Hold for five seconds.
3   Breathe out for five seconds.
4   Hold for five seconds.
5   Repeat.

NATURAL REMEDIES FOR SLEEP

Some individuals may resort to nutritional supplements to aid sleep, including magnesium, valerian root, or lemon balm:

Magnesium is an essential mineral that has been shown to improve sleep quality. Most adults in the UK do not consume the correct levels required by our bodies (375 mg per day), and this may interfere with our sleep. Magnesium can be incorporated in meals by ingesting green leafy vegetables.

Valerian root has been used since the ancient Greeks and Romans. According to the Sleep Foundation, it contains multiple chemical compounds known to impact serotonin receptors as well as reduce brain activity in the motor cortex. Studies have shown that Valerian root supplements helps people fall asleep faster, improve their sleep quality, and spend more time in the deep-sleep stage.

Lemon balm taken as a supplement has been found in studies to reduce symptoms of insomnia in 42% of a young and healthy population.

It should be noted that taking any supplements should be checked out with healthcare professionals, as they may interfere with other medications you are taking.

WHITE NOISE

Some noises are said to stimulate our brain and disrupt sleep, such as car horns and barking dogs, whilst other noises can relax our brain and promote better sleep, such as white noise. **White noise** is defined as noise that contains a mixture of all audible frequencies that human ears can hear. Pure white noise is said to resemble a 'hissy shhh' sound. Studies indicate that listening to white noise is a good sleep aid as it blocks out other sounds that can startle us out of sleep. It is also believed that white noise may assist individuals when studying and experiencing stress. But have you heard of brown noise, pink noise, and even black noise?

White noise – Examples include the sounds of whirring fans, radio or television static, crackling and hissing sounds, and humming air conditioners.

Brown noise (also called **red noise**) – Deeper and softer than pink or white noise. Examples include low roaring, powerful waterfalls, and thunder.

Pink noise – White noise but with reduced higher frequencies and therefore less harsh. Nature is full of pink noise, including rustling leaves, steady rain, wind, heartbeats, and ocean waves. Pink noise is said to be the best to aid sleep.

Black noise – An informal term used to describe a lack of noise: either complete silence or very little noise.

Noise types get their names based on colours of light wavelengths (see Chapter 8). You can listen to these noises on your computer or smartphone or a specialised sleep machine like a white noise machine.

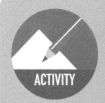

Chapter 3 Activity

This is a good exercise for helping induce sleep – a modern take on counting sheep:

Take a moment or two to get yourself comfortable in bed, lying down. Take a deep breath in, pause, and then exhale slowly. Feel how you sink down into the bed.

Open your mouth wide, and let your jaw drop. Then wiggle your toes and feel your feet and legs, hands, and arms – move them a little if you wish.

Take another deep breath in, and feel any tension in your chest and stomach before exhaling out slowly. Spend a moment or two focusing on your body and relaxing any areas of tension.

Now to begin the sleep countdown: with each number you count, allow yourself to feel more and more relaxed and drowsy.

Count very slowly, breathe with each count, and focus on the countdown and the numbers. Thoughts may invade your mind; acknowledge them and then let them go, turning your attention back on the numbers.

Starting with **50**, breathe in, and silently count 50. Picture the number **50**. Then breathe out to the number **50**.

Picture the number **49**. Breathe in and then breath out to the number **49**.

Picture the number **48**. Breathe in and then breath out to the number **48**. Feel your eyelids becoming heavier.

Picture the number **47**. Breathe in and then breath out to the number **47**.

Picture the number **46**. Breathe in and then breath out to the number **46**.

Picture the number **45**. Breathe in and then breath out to the number **45**. Focus all your attention on the number **45**.

Picture the number **44**. Breathe in and then breath out to the number **44**.

Picture the number **43**. Breathe in and then breath out to the number **43**. All is calm and peaceful.

Picture the number **42**. Breathe in and then breath out to the number **42**. If your attention drifts, focus on the number.

Picture the number **41**. Breathe in and then breath out to the number **41**. You are beginning to feel more relaxed and sleepy.

Picture the number **40**. Breathe in and then breath out to the number **40**. You are calm, and everything is peaceful.

Picture the number **39**. Breathe in and then breath out to the number **39**.

Picture the number **38**. Breathe in and then breath out to the number **38**. Deeply relaxed. Deeper and deeper.

Picture the number **37**. Breathe in and then breath out to the number **37**.

Picture the number **36**. Breathe in and then breath out to the number **36**. Calm and relaxed.

Picture the number **35**. Breathe in and then breath out to the number **35**.

Picture the number **34**. Breathe in and then breath out to the number **34**. Slowly counting down to sleep.

Picture the number **33**. Breathe in and then breath out to the number **33**.

Picture the number **32**. Breathe in and then breath out to the number **32**. Peaceful and relaxed.

Picture the number **31**. Breathe in and then breath out to the number **31**.

Picture the number **30**. Breathe in and then breath out to the number **30**.

Continue to count down on your own, all the way down to zero. Deep down to sleep.

KEY POINTS

- Sleepless nights
- Sleep schedules
- The benefits of a good night's sleep
- Worrying about not getting enough sleep
- Equation for how well you sleep
- Orthosomnia remedies

- Military sleep technique
- Sleep deprivation
- The paradoxical sleep technique
- Clean sleeping
- Working night shifts
- Shift work sleep disorder
- Complications of shift work sleep disorder
- Shift work sleep disorder treatment
- White noise

WEB RESOURCES

NHS Sleep: https://www.nhs.uk/live-well/sleep-and-tiredness/

Cambridge University Sleep Study: http://www.pressreader.com/uk/daily-record/20220429/281973201222016

Paradoxical sleep hack: https://www.powerofpositivity.com/fall-asleep-fast-hack/

Circadian rhythm: https://www.sleepfoundation.org/circadian-rhythm

Equation for how well you sleep: https://www.dailymail.co.uk/health/article-2454082/sleep-quality-equation-works-sleep-improve-it

Sleep deprivation: https://www.health.com/mind-body/signs-of-sleep-deprivation

Clean sleeping: http://www.hollandandbarrett.com/the-health-hub/conditions/sleep/sleep-help/what-is-clean-sleeping

Shift work disorder: http://www.sleepfoundation.org/sleep-disorders/shift-work-disorder

Foods and sleep deprivation: https://www.msn.com/en-gb/health/nutrition/sleep-deprivation-the-effects-and-the-foods-that-could-help/ss-AA12xaKW

White noise: https://www.healthline.com/health/pink-noise-sleep#other-sleeping-tips

PART 2
• • • • • • • • • • • • • • • • • • • •
STRATEGIES
TO COMBAT
STRESS

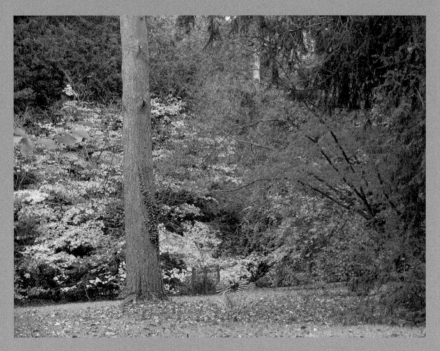

Chapter 4

BREATHING THERAPY

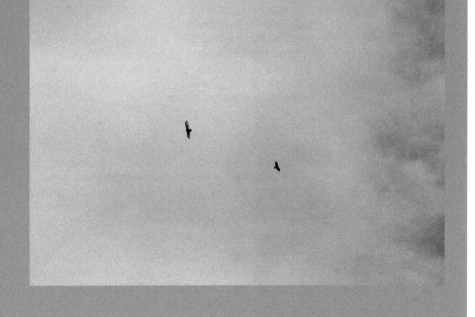

Wellbeing Strategies for Nurses, First Edition. Claire Boyd.
© 2023 John Wiley & Sons Ltd. Published 2023 by John Wiley & Sons Ltd.

LEARNING OUTCOMES

By the end of this chapter, you will have an understanding of the health benefits of learning deep-breathing techniques and the bodily responses to stress and breathing patterns.

Stress and our breathing patterns are interlinked. When we are stressed, our respiratory rate, blood pressure, and heart rate increase due to the release of a hormone called corticotropin-releasing hormone (CRH) by the hypothalamus. One of the simplest things we can all do to manage our stress is to breathe deeply. This is because an anxious person typically takes rapid and shallow breaths, using their shoulders rather than the diaphragm to move the air in and out of the lungs. This style of breathing disrupts the balance of gases in the body. Breathing through your chest creates a stressful experience for your body and communicates to your brain that you are not in a relaxed state. To rectify this situation, you will need to work on inhaling and exhaling using the diaphragm: take 6–10 deep abdominal breaths for 10 minutes. This will reduce your heart rate by 15–20 beats per minute and, at the same time, decrease your respiratory rate by 20–30%. If you have the time, continue this exercise for 20 minutes for the best results.

HOW DOES IT WORK?

Breathing techniques have long been used in traditional relaxation techniques, such as yoga and meditation, as well as the more modern relaxation techniques advocating the importance of taking deep breaths. The immediate impact of doing this can be seen in the reduced production of two stress hormones: noradrenaline and cortisol.

Research by scientists at Stanford University has identified a group of nerves in our brains called the **pre-Bötzinger complex** that regulates our breathing. The scientists found that changes in the expression of certain genes in these nerves – which are physically connected to critical areas in the brain associated with relaxation, attention, excitement, and panic – can calm an individual. The implication is that changes in breathing directly affect stress levels.

HYPERVENTILATION

We all may worry about our finances (or lack of), difficulty sleeping, feeling overwhelmed at work, and/or being unable to switch off. The worst-case scenario may result in us being so overwhelmed that hyperventilation occurs.

Hyperventilation can make us feel like we are not getting enough oxygen into our body, causing us to gasp for breath. We may experience:

- Dizziness
- Feeling faint
- Feeling lightheaded
- Tingling in the fingers

During hyperventilation, when we feel we are not getting enough oxygen, we try to take deeper, more rapid breaths. But in fact, we are getting **too much** oxygen and making the situation worse by taking these deeper, rapid breaths. Since the problem is caused by an overabundance of oxygen and not enough carbon dioxide, the hyperventilation can get worse, causing:

- Worsening lightheadedness
- Chest pain
- Leg/extremity weakness
- Palpitations/tachycardia

Focusing on your breathing will help to reset the breathing pattern.

HEALTH BENEFITS OF DEEP BREATHING

Deep breathing releases toxins from the body. Up to 70% of the toxins that the body retains are meant to be expelled through the breathing process. If you are breathing deeply and performing this practice more often, you can expel these toxins more effectively. The primary toxin that is expelled through the breathing process is carbon dioxide. When we exhale after a deep breath, we remove the carbon dioxide that has been produced from our metabolism activities.

The carbon dioxide is in our blood, which is then oxygenated by the lungs, and the oxygen is deposited in its place.

Deep Breathing Reduces Stress and Muscular Tension

A deep breath is also a message that is sent to the rest of the body. It's a way of telling the brain that it is time to slow down and relax for a minute. As this message spreads throughout the body, a feeling of calmness begins to settle in. Tense muscles start to ease. Anxiety may begin to fade.

Cortisol is known as the stress hormone because it is usually produced only in situations which are considered to be personally stressful. By reducing the amount of stress being felt, it is possible for daily deep breathing exercises to manage stress-related health problems with greater effectiveness. This can mean a reduction in the risk of heart disease symptoms, stroke, hypertension, and even diabetes.

Deep Breathing Can Control Chronic Pain

When we experience pain, we tend to tense up and breath through the chest (shallow breathing), disrupting the balance of oxygen and carbon dioxide in the body, which may further aggravate the pain. By learning to 'deep breathe' using the diaphragm, we can actually hep to reduce the pain. This process works effectively to manage acute or chronic pain because deep breathing causes the body to release endorphins. Endorphins help your body feel better because they stimulate the mind's reward centres.

Deep Breathing Can Reduce Incidents of Insomnia

There are a lot of stimulants in what we eat and drink. It is not just caffeine that can keep us awake at night. If we consume something that contains a high level of sugar, there is a good chance we'll have difficulty sleeping. Deep breathing is known to counter the effects of stimulants on the central nervous system. The deep-breathing process helps create relaxation, which means the nervous system does not feel as 'amped up' by the stimulants.

Deep breathing is also important because the process can help quiet the mind. It is much easier to fall asleep and then stay asleep when the mind is clear and calm. Deep breathing can have an immediate impact.

Deep Breathing Can Help with Migraines

Migraine headaches can be very debilitating. Migraine sufferers may experience dizziness, nausea, photophobia, and/or a slower thinking process. Some migraines last a short while, whilst others can continue for hours. The start of a migraine can create muscle tension in the face, neck, and shoulders, enhancing the pain of the migraine. Deep breathing alone generally will not get rid of a migraine, as a multifaceted approach is needed, such as taking medications and avoiding migraine triggers (smoke, perfume, certain foods, etc.);– but one part of the treatment plan for migraines includes deep breathing. This is because it boosts the blood circulated to the brain so the body can begin healing naturally.

Deep Breathing Works with Brainwave-Entrainment Products

Some programs used for relaxation and meditation include deep breathing, such as taking a warm, scented bath or shower or listening to white noise.

Deep Breathing Can Change the Acidity Level of the Body

Deep breathing helps make the body more alkaline than acidic. This lowering of the pH also helps control pain because the receptors related to pain respond more quickly to internal responses. When we are stressed out, pain tends to be worse because cortisol is a pain conductor and amplifies what we feel. Deep breathing reduces the amount of cortisol in the body – even chronic pain can be lessened.

Deep Breathing Exercises Are Encouraged in Many Practices in Life

From meditation to birthing, the way we breathe can have an immediate positive impact on personal health.

SIMPLE BREATHING TECHNIQUES

Although we all breathe, some of us may have learnt poor breathing patterns, which can be easily rectified by learning to take slower, deeper breaths. In the following exercises, we will look at 13 breathing exercises, all of which take just a few minutes to perform and can be done anywhere – standing up, sitting in a chair with your feet on the ground, or lying on a bed or on the floor on a yoga mat! Most of these techniques have their foundations in yoga.

You will get the most benefit if you practise the techniques regularly. Find the technique that you like the best and that works for you. Note that you should not try all these breathing techniques in one sitting – pace them out. Let's start with an instant fix.

EXERCISE 4.1   For Instant Calm

This is an NHS breathing exercise to relieve stress:

1   Either sitting or standing, place both feet flat on the ground roughly hip-width apart.
2   Let your breath flow as deep into your abdomen as is comfortable, without forcing it.
3   Breath in through your nose and out through your mouth.
4   Breathe in gently and regularly. You may find it useful to count steadily from 1 to 5. You may not be able to reach 5 at first.
5   Then, without pausing or holding your breath, let it flow out gently, counting from 1 to 5 again.
6   Keep doing this for three to five minutes.

STUDENT TIP

When practising this deep-breathing technique, I don't count but slowly sing in my mind the song by the Police:

Inhaling: 'every breath you take'

Pause: 'and every move you make'

Exhale: 'I'll be watching you'

As you get better at it, you can add on 'Every bond you break, every step you take' when you exhale.

Note that you should not force any of these breathing techniques. As you practice them, deep breathing exercises will strengthen the lungs over time.

EXERCISE 4.2   Diaphragmatic Breathing Technique

This technique enables us to re-establish diaphragmatic breathing rather than shoulder breathing. Diaphragmatic breathing is a good technique to use before stressful events such as exams or other situations that cause anxiety:

1   Sit comfortably.
2   Place one hand on your stomach just below the navel and the other on your chest.
3   Close your eyes to cut out extraneous stimuli.
4   Breathe in deeply and slowly through the nose, silently counting to 4.
5   Slowly exhale through the mouth, again counting to 4.
6   Try to make your diaphragm (abdomen area) rise and fall, keeping your chest and shoulders still.
7   While breathing in, visualise warm air flowing into all parts of your body.
8   While breathing out, imagine that the tension and stress are leaving.

EXERCISE 4.3   The Sedona Method

This breathing technique helps to let go of stress and worry. It is a method that is said to give you the power to address the issues that you need to be free of by 'releasing them'.

This method is a bit too hippie for me, but it may work for you, so I felt the need to include it:

1   Think of an issue that is causing you anxiety.
2   Welcome it. Allow it to be present as you fully come to terms with how it affects you and how it makes you feel.
3   Now, take a deep breath and ask yourself these three questions:
Do I want to let go of the emotions bubbling up from this issue?
Can I let the emotions around this issue go?
When do I want to let these emotions go?

4   Answer as truthfully as possible. The answers to the first two questions should be a simple 'Yes' or 'No'. You should not allow other thoughts to interfere, such as justifying holding on to the feeling.

5   When the answer to the third question is 'Now', release your breath, and feel the tension melt away.

6   If your answers to questions 1 and 2 are 'no', that's OK. Ask the question again until you feel ready to let go.

DID YOU KNOW?

Sedona is in Arizona, USA. It is a mecca for healers where a variety of shamanic traditions can be found, including Native Americans, Andean (South America), and Mayan (Mexico). Many western teachers have worked with native medicine men and women where these traditions originated and adapted these practices to complement conventional (allopathic) medicine.

EXERCISE 4.4   Equal Breathing Technique

This is a good technique to use at night if you struggle to fall asleep after a hectic day:

1   When you feel stressed, inhale through your nose to a count of 4.
2   Now exhale through your nose to a count of 4.
3   Each time you inhale and exhale, keep in mind your goal to calm yourself and rid your body of tension.
4   Keep this sequence up for six cycles.

EXERCISE 4.5   Moon Breath or Left-Nostril Breathing

This Japanese breathing technique is good for calming the mind and promoting sleep. The left side of the body is thought to be associated with the nervous system, so it has long been used in stress relief:

1 Lie down, and close your eyes.
2 Use your right thumb to gently close your right nostril and restrict the airflow.
3 Breathe naturally through the left nostril, making sure air flows without restriction. Then close it using your finger, and breathe out through your right nostril.
4 Inhale and exhale slowly for a few minutes this way. You should start to feel peace and calm.

EXERCISE 4.6   Ocean Breathing Technique

This technique is good for balancing the body to relieve tension and anxiety:

1 Sit with your back upright, and close your eyes. Breathe deeply in and out through your nose.
2 As you inhale and exhale, constrict the muscles in your throat to produce a whooshing sound.
3 When you breathe in this manner, the air should pass smoothly through your throat, and your throat should feel as natural as possible.
4 Balance the power of each breath as you inhale and exhale. Balance the sounds of your breaths.

DID YOU KNOW?

Deep breathing can help with acute and chronic pain due to the 'distraction strategy' - taking your mind away from the pain due to concentrating hard on the deep breathing technique/process.

EXERCISE 4.7   Pursed-LIP Breathing

This technique slows the pace of your breathing by having you apply deliberate effort with each breath. You can practice pursed-lip breathing at any time. It may be especially useful during activities such as bending, lifting, or climbing stairs. Think of weight-lifters during the Olympics who use this technique:

1 Relax your neck and shoulders.
2 Keep your mouth closed, and inhale slowly through your nose for a count of 2.
3 Pucker or purse your lips as though you are about to whistle.
4 Exhale slowly by blowing air through your pursed lips for a count of 4.

EXERCISE 4.8   Lion's Breath

Lion's breath is an energising yoga breathing practice that is said to relieve tension in your chest and face. Note: This breathing technique needs to be performed in private unless you wish to scare people!

1   Sit comfortably in a chair or on the floor with crossed legs (if you can manage this).
2   Press your palms down against your knees with your fingers spread wide.
3   Inhale deeply through your nose, and open your eyes wide – really make them pop!
4   At the same time, open your mouth wide and stick out your tongue, bringing the tip down towards your chin. (Think of the Maori haka performed before rugby matches!)
5   Contract the muscles at the front of your throat as you exhale out through your mouth, making a long 'ha' sound.
6   You can turn your gaze to look at the space between your eyebrows or the tip of your nose.
7   Do this two to three times.

EXERCISE 4.9   Humming Bee Breath

This is another yoga technique that helps to create instant calm. Individuals tend to use humming bee breaths to relieve frustration, anxiety, and even anger, so it's great to use after dealing with tricky visitors or patients!

1   Get into a comfortable seated position.
2   Close your eyes, and relax your face.
3   Place your index fingers on the tragus cartilage that partially covers your ear canal.
4   Inhale, and as you exhale, gently press your fingers into the cartilage.
5   Keeping your mouth closed, make a loud humming sound.
6   Continue for as long as comfortable.

EXERCISE 4.10   7-11 Breathing Technique

This technique is especially good when you are stressed due to an anxiety-provoking situation, like before an exam or an interview, and you may start to hyperventilate. There is a deliberate longer count on the out breath to reverse the effects of the hyperventilation. If you practice this breathing technique when you feel fine, it will be easier to use in an emergency:

1   Breathe in for a count of 7 and out for a count of 11. Don't worry if you count quickly; you will get better over time.
2   Repeat until you start to feel calmer.

EXERCISE 4.11   Resonant Breathing

This technique involves breathing at a rate of five full breaths per minute. You achieve this rate by inhaling and exhaling for a count of 5. Breathing at this rate maximises your heart rate variability (HRV), reduces stress, and, according to a 2017 study, can reduce symptoms of depression when combined with a yoga technique called Iyengar:

1   Inhale for a count of 5.
2   Exhale for a count of 5.
3   Continue this breathing pattern for at least a few minutes.

EXERCISE 4.12   Breath Focus Technique

This deep breathing technique uses focus words:

1   Sit or lie down in a comfortable place.
2   Bring your awareness to your breaths without trying to change how you're breathing.
3   Alternate between normal and deep breaths a few times. Notice any differences between normal breathing and deep breathing. Notice how your abdomen expands with deep inhalation.
4   Note how shallow breathing feels compared to deep breathing.
5   Practice your deep breathing for a few minutes.
6   Place one hand below your belly button, keeping your abdomen relaxed, and notice how it rises with each inhale and falls with each exhale.
7   Let out a loud sigh with each exhale.
8   Begin the practice of breath focus by combining this deep breathing with a focus word or phrase that will support relaxation.
9   You can imagine that the air you inhale brings waves of peace and calm throughout your body. Mentally say 'inhaling peace and calm'.
10 Imagine that the air you exhale washes away tension and anxiety. You can say to yourself, 'exhaling tension and anxiety'.

EXERCISE 4.13   4-7-8 Breathing Technique

The 4-7-8 breathing technique is a breathing pattern developed by Dr Andrew Weil. It is based on an ancient yogic technique called **pranayama**, and it actually helps you to gain control over your breathing.

Using the 4-7-8 breathing techniques activates your parasympathetic nervous system (responsible for relaxation). When you activate this system, your body suppresses the opposite system (the sympathetic nervous system), which is responsible for the stress response – the fight-or-flight reaction.

This breathing technique can be used to calm your anxiety in the moment, but it is said to work better as a daily preventative practice. Using this breathing practice regularly helps you control your own breath, helping to make the voluntary aspect involuntary.

You can use the ratio 4-7-8 (exhaling longer than inhaling):

- At work, when experiencing stress
- When driving to or from work whilst stuck in traffic
- During exams or interviews
- At night when trying to fall asleep
- Before giving a speech or presentation
- When feeling overwhelmed, anxious, or stressed
- When you first wake up in the morning

Studies have found that the benefits of the 4-7-8 breathing technique (as with other deep breathing exercises) include:

- Reduced depression and anxiety
- Improved sleep quality
- Reduced stress levels
- Improved motor memory
- Improved pain processing

This breathing exercise is best performed sitting rather than lying down. Try not to focus on other thoughts during the practice – keep all your focus and attention on your breath. To perform the exercise:

1   Sit down, and put one hand on your chest and another on your stomach area.
2   Close your mouth, and inhale through your nose – take a deep, slow breath from your stomach, counting to 4 as you breath in.
3   Hold your breath completely and slowly while silently counting from 1 to 7.
4   Release your breath slowly and completely through your mouth whilst silently counting from 1 to 8.
5   Repeat three to seven times or until you feel calm.

Chapter 4 Activity

In this activity, we look at fun breathing techniques. These techniques were initially developed for children – find your inner child, and have a go at these breathing exercises:

 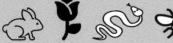

Smelling flowers – Imagine you are smelling a flower, breathing in deeply
 through your nose and out through your mouth.
The bunny breath – Just like a bunny, take three quick sniffs through your nose
 and one long exhale out through your nose.
Blow out the candles – Imagine blowing out the candles on a make-believe
 birthday cake, drawing a deep breath in through your mouth and blowing it
 out through your mouth as well.
The snake breath – Inhale deeply through your nose and blow out through your
 mouth with a soft, low hissing sound.
Blow bubbles – Imagine softly blowing a nice big bubble. Take a breath in, and
 blow it out soft and long.
Smell the flower and blow out the candle – Imagine you have a flower in one
 hand and a candle in the other. Smell the flower: take a deep breath in
 through your nose, and fill the lungs with air. Then exhale and blow out the
 candle in your other hand.
Bumblebee breath – Inhale through your nose, keeping your mouth closed. With
 your mouth still closed, make a humming or buzzing noise (like a bumblebee)
 as you exhale.
Dragonfly breath – Interlace your fingers under your chin and, as you inhale,
 raise your elbows as high as you can around your neck and face. On the
 exhale, lower your elbows back down.
Hot-air-balloon breath – Cup your hands around your mouth. Inhale deeply. On
 the exhale (through your mouth), expand your hands outward as if you are
 blowing up a giant hot air balloon.
Shoulder-roll breath – This breathing exercise has the added benefit of releasing
 tight muscles and tension. As you take a deep breath in, roll your shoulders
 up towards your ears. Then drop your shoulders back down on the exhale.

KEY POINTS

- Bodily responses to stress and breathing patterns
- The benefits of learning breathing techniques
- Hyperventilation
- Health benefits of deep breathing
- 13 breathing techniques
- Fun breathing exercises

WEB RESOURCES

- **Breathing techniques:** https://www.nhs.uk/mental-health/self-help/guides-tools-and-activities/breathing-exercises-for-stress/
- **Breathing exercises:** https://www.verywellhealth.com/how-to-do-deep-breathing-exercises-1945350, https://adrenalfatiguesolution.com/5-simple-breathing-exercises/, https://positivepsychology.com/deep-breathing-techniques-exercises
- **Breathing exercises for children/fun:** https://www.moshikids.com/articles/deep-breathing-exercises-for-kids
- **Moon breathing:** https://www.elle.com/uk/beauty/body-and-physical-health/a29544671/moon-breathing-sleep-insomnia

Chapter 5
MUSCLE RELAXATION

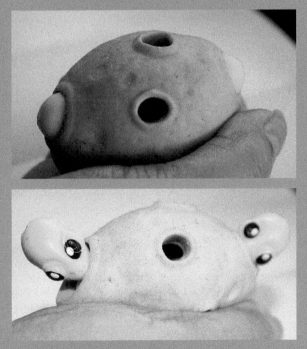

Wellbeing Strategies for Nurses, First Edition. Claire Boyd.
© 2023 John Wiley & Sons Ltd. Published 2023 by John Wiley & Sons Ltd.

This chapter looks at muscle tensing and relaxing to release the tension you may be carrying. To be honest, If I squeezed a stress ball and two little aliens popped out, like in the picture, I would be quite stressed! And just to note, no aliens were harmed in making this photo.

PROGRESSIVE MUSCLE RELAXATION

Progressive muscle relaxation (commonly called PMR) is a technique whereby the muscles in the body are tensed and then released, helping the body to progressively relax. This technique is used to decrease muscle tension, fatigue, neck and back pain, and even muscle spasms.

BRIEF HISTORY OF PMR

PMR was first described by the American physician Edmund Jacobson in 1908 at Harvard University. In 1929, the book *Progressive Relaxation* described this technique used to remove muscular tension – a method of deep muscle relaxation. It is a technique of tightening and systematically loosening muscle groups throughout the body and is one of the most commonly used relaxation techniques for stress relief in healthcare today.

I often begin my relaxation sessions with this muscle tense-and-release exercise. It could be by focusing on specific muscle areas of the body or by doing an exercise like imagining you are a piece of seaweed, ebbing and flowing with the waves.

The following exercise teaches how to recognise and reduce muscle tension, especially if you are new to this technique. You can relieve tension in any part of the body just by tensing and relaxing each muscle in turn.

EXERCISE 5.1   Reducing Muscle Tension

1 Close your eyes, and concentrate on your breathing.
2 Slowly breathe in through your nose and out through your mouth.
3 Now make a fist with your hand, squeezing your hand tightly.
4 Hold for a few seconds, noticing the tension.
5 Slowly open your fingers, and feel the difference – notice the tension leaving. Your hand should feel much lighter and more relaxed.
6 Perform this exercise again with the other hand.

WHAT ARE THE BENEFITS OF PMR?

PMR helps us to distinguish between tensed muscles and relaxed ones so that we can rectify the problem; it also helps the whole body progressively relax. This technique can reduce physiological tension caused by worry and anxiety.

WHAT EVIDENCE IS THERE THAT PMR WORKS?

Science has recognised the benefits of PMR in a range of fields:

Health – PMR is so successful in healthcare settings, along with other relaxation techniques, that it is offered by many medical practitioners to patients such as those with depression and stress-related issues and sleep disorders.

Sport – PMR is used in sports for competitive athletes experiencing anxiety preparing for events.

Oncology – Studies have shown that PMR offers some relief in those undertaking chemotherapy, reducing symptoms of pain, nausea, anxiety, and depression in cancer patients.

Education – PMR has proved successful in the learning environment. Students using the technique are found to have increased mental and physical relaxation and lowered stress levels.

TENSION AND RELAXATION

There are two basic parts to PMR, as seen in Table 5.1.

Table 5.1 Recognition and relaxation.

The recognition of tension in muscles	This is where we check for tension in each muscle group in the body. Major tension areas include the shoulders, jaw, and forehead. Since there is tension in every muscle group, progression in a logical order is required to recognise and alleviate this tension.
The relaxation of each muscle group	As you focus on a muscle group, the relaxation process can begin by tensing the muscle, holding the tension for a few seconds, and then relaxing the muscle slowly for a few seconds. You should feel the tension draining from the body. This tensing and relaxing of the muscles can be repeated several times before moving on to the next muscle group.

PMR EXERCISES

There are many variations of the PMR technique, and we will look at three adaptations, starting with a basic one for beginners. It is a good idea to read the script first and record it on your phone so that it can be played back during the exercise.

Throughout the exercises, breathe at a nice steady rate. To begin, either get comfortable in a chair or lie on the floor. Anyone with a medical condition should check first with their general practitioner to be sure they can undertake these PMR exercises.

EXERCISE 5.2   PMR Exercise for Beginners

Put on some soothing music at a low volume. Remove your shoes. Lie comfortably on the floor in a quiet room with a cushion under your head for support. You can start at the head/face or toes. Perform the exercise slowly.
(20 MINUTES)

1   Focus on your breathing.
    Slowly breathe in and out, emphasising the out breath.
    Take a few more breaths before moving on.
2   Tense the muscles in your right foot, hold for a few seconds, and then release.
    Tense and release the calf muscle and then the thigh muscles (tense and release).

Repeat with the left foot and leg.
3   Tense and release the muscles in your right hand.
    Tense and release the muscles in your right arm.
    Then the left hand and arm.
4   Tense and release each buttock.
    Then the stomach muscles.
5   Lift your shoulders up to your ears, hold for a few seconds, and then lower. Repeat three times.
    Rock your head gently from side to side.
6   Yawn – then pout. Frown, wrinkle your nose, and let go.
    Raise your eyebrows, and then relax your face muscles.
7   Focus on your breathing again. Wriggle your fingers and toes, bend your knees, gently roll over onto your side, and then get up slowly.

EXERCISE 5.3   PMR Variation 1

This exercise has a slight twist to the tensing-and-relaxing PMR technique. It is important to remember that the more you practice PMR, the more relaxed you will feel performing the exercise.

Muscle group	Action
Hands	Clench/make a fist. Relax.
Shoulders	Shrug them (raise them towards your ears). Relax.
Forehead	Wrinkle into a deep frown. Relax.
Eyes and nose	Close your eyes as tightly as possible. Relax. Note: If you wear contact lenses, you may need to remove them before the start of this exercise.
Cheeks and jaws	Smile as widely as you can – think Cheshire Cat! Relax.
Mouth	Press your lips together tightly. Check your face for tension. Relax.

(Continued)

Muscle group	Action
Back of neck	Press the back of your head against your support (chair headrest or the floor). Relax.
Front of neck	Touch your chin to your chest. Relax.
Chest	Take a deep breath, and hold for 5–10 seconds. Relax.
Back	Arch your back up and away from the floor or chair. Relax.
Stomach	Suck in your stomach. Relax.
Hips and buttocks	Press your buttocks together tightly. Relax.
Thighs	Clench your thighs. Relax.
Lower legs	Point your toes towards your face. Then point your toes away and curl them downward at the same time. Relax.

EXERCISE 5.4   PMR Variation 2

During this exercise, you will probably feel heavy at the start and lighter at the end if you have achieved relaxation.

Muscle group	Action
1 Right foot and lower leg	Keeping the heel down, curl the toes back until tension can be felt in your ankle and calf muscles. Relax.
2 Right upper leg	Tense the top of your upper leg (quadriceps) and the bottom of your upper leg (hamstring). Relax.
3 Left foot, lower leg, and upper leg	Repeat steps 1 and 2. Relax.

Muscle group	Action
4 Right hand and forearm	With the palm down, lift your hand until tension can be felt in the top of the hand, the wrist, and the forearm. Relax.
5 Right upper arm	Tense your bicep and tricep. Relax.
6 Right shoulder	Shrug your shoulder towards your ear, and roll your head towards your shoulder so that the shoulder and ear are touching. Relax.
7 Left hand and forearm, upper arm, and shoulder	Repeat steps 4, 5, and 6. Relax.
8 Jaw area	Without damaging your teeth, bite down until tension can be felt in the jaw area. Relax.
9 Mouth	Purse your lips as if you are whistling. Relax.
10 Chin	Place the bottom of your tongue on the roof of your mouth, and push upward. Relax.
11 Forehead	Wrinkle your brow. Relax.

Instead of tensing your muscles, another variation of a muscle-relaxing exercise is to place something warm (not hot) on each part of your body in turn.

MUSCLE RELAXATION

Just as there are variations of the PMR exercise, there are also other ways we can relax our tense and/or aching muscles, especially if we have been on our feet all shift. Exercises 5.5 and 5.6 shows two bath exercises to enjoy – one for the feet and one for the body.

EXERCISE 5.5   Foot Bath

If you have been on your feet all day, a good way to relieve aches and pains is to have a nice foot bath. Add four to six drops of rosemary essential oil to a bowl of warm water, and soak your feet for 10 minutes.

EXERCISE 5.6   Epsom Bath

Adding Epsom salts to a warm bath makes you feel more lightweight and buoyant while helping your muscles to relax. Your body also absorbs the salts, which helps replenish magnesium stores, a mineral that is reduced when you feel stressed.

RELIEVING TENSION WITH DISTRACTION

Another way to relieve tension from the body is by using distraction. The next exercise shows how colour, creativity, and movement can help you feel relaxed, releasing tension by:

- Distracting you from worrying thoughts
- Giving you an outlet to focus your emotions
- Stimulating your senses.

EXERCISE 5.7   Draw Calming Circles

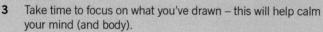

1   Make sure you are sitting comfortably with your feet firmly on the ground, your back straight, and your shoulders relaxed.
2   Take a coloured pencil and some paper, and draw a circle. Try not to let your pencil leave the page – keep creating lots of circles.
3   Take time to focus on what you've drawn – this will help calm your mind (and body).
4   Once you have done this for a few minutes, choose another coloured pencil and create more circles.

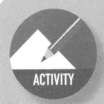

Chapter 5 Activity

ACTIVITY

Tension Relief Bath

This is similar to the PMR exercise for releasing tension from the muscle groups, but it has the added benefit of a warm scented bath.

1   Run a warm bath. Add 12 drops of lavender essential oil, and swish the water around. Get into the bath. Close your eyes, and spend a moment enjoying the warm water on your body and the soothing smell of the lavender oil.

2   Lift your arms in the air, bending them at the elbow and clenching your fists. Breathe in deeply. As you breathe out, release your clenched fists. Lower your arms gently, and imagine the tension in them draining away into the water.

3   Now shrug your shoulders as high as you can. Feel the tension in your head, shoulders, neck, and chest. Hold for a moment, and then, on the out breath, slowly release and lower your shoulders. Imagine the tension flowing away into the water.

4   Tighten your facial muscles by screwing up your face and clenching your teeth. Hold for a few seconds and then let go.

5   Continue working through your muscles, tensing and releasing this way, paying particular attention to your back, abdomen, buttocks, and legs.

At the end, a feeling of calmness and relaxation should wash over you.

KEY POINTS

- Progressive muscle relaxation (PMR)
- Brief history of PMR
- Benefits of PMR
- Evidence that PMR works
- PMR key components: recognition and relaxation
- PMR exercise for beginners
- PMR variations 1 and 2
- Other methods of muscle relaxation
- Using distraction for tension relief

WEB RESOURCES

Muscle relaxation: https://www.sciencedirect.com/topics/
medicine-and-dentistry/progressive-muscle-relaxation
Relaxation: www.mind.org.uk/information-support/tips-for-
everyday-living/relaxation/relaxation-exercises

Chapter 6

· · · · · · · · · · · · · · · · · · ·

NATURE (BIOPHILIA THEORY)

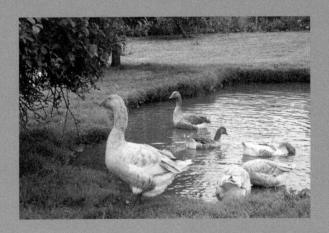

Wellbeing Strategies for Nurses, First Edition. Claire Boyd.
© 2023 John Wiley & Sons Ltd. Published 2023 by John Wiley & Sons Ltd.

LEARNING OUTCOMES

By the end of this chapter, you will have an understanding of the therapeutic benefits of nature for wellbeing, the biophilia hypothesis, how to connect with nature, and the benefits of shinrin-yoku (Forest bathing).

A number of studies have highlighted the therapeutic benefits of green and blue spaces. What are green and blue spaces, you may ask? **Green spaces** are defined as open, undeveloped land with natural vegetation, whilst **blue spaces** are defined as visible surface water, such as lakes, rivers, or coastal waters and also urban water like canals or ponds.

Doctors and psychologists 'prescribe nature' to improve mental health in patients, and many schools in the UK have 'forest schools': sessions away from the classroom, in woodlands, parks, etc., providing opportunities for children to learn about nature, run and let off steam, and have opportunities for calm reflection, improving their psychological wellbeing. Listening to birdsong and observing animals in nature has been shown to promote wellbeing, reduce stress, improve mood, and reduce attention fatigue. Natural aromas from woods and plants have calming effects, and viewing nature reduces mental fatigue.

HEALTH BENEFITS OF NATURE

Studies suggest that some of the health benefits of spending time in nature include:

- Increasing happiness and improving mood
- Reducing stress and anger
- Helping those who have anxiety and depression
- Helping those experiencing SAD (seasonal affective disorder)
- Boosting relaxation
- Encouraging you learn new skills (some research even suggests it makes you smarter)
- Helping you feel more connected to nature, yourself, and other people

DID YOU KNOW?

Going into a green space can actually be quite stressful if you are being chased in a field by a bull! LOL

The National Park Service in the USA suggests that nature makes you smarter, stronger, healthier, and more productive (see Table 6.1).

THE BIOPHILIA HYPOTHESIS

The **biophilia hypothesis** suggests that humans have a tendency to focus on and affiliate with nature and other life forms due in part to genetics, meaning the human brain evolved in a biocentric world.

Table 6.1 Benefits of nature according to the US National Park Service.

Smarter	Just 20 minutes in nature improves concentration and reduces the need for ADHD (attention deficit hyperactivity disorder) and ADD (attention deficit disorder) medications in children. Walking through nature can greatly improve performance in school by improving cognitive function and memory. Physical activity in a green space can reduce stress and lower cortisol levels by 15%.
Stronger	Exercising in nature leads to greater health benefits than performing the same activity indoors. Communities closer to nature are more likely to have stronger ties with their community members.
Healthier	A 30-minute visit to a park can improve heart health and circulation and lower cholesterol, blood glucose, and blood pressure. Walking in nature boosts your immune system, which decreases the risk of certain diseases and cancers.
Happier	Five minutes of walking in nature improves mood, self-esteem, and relaxation. Frequent exposure to nature reduces anxiety and depression whilst promoting a sense of wellbeing and fulfilment.
More productive	Physical activity in a green space can improve cognitive control, short- and long-term memory, and overall brain function. Children who walk 20 minutes in a park concentrate longer in school.

Research evidence suggests that humans are innately attracted to nature, with its rich diversity of shapes, colours, textures, and life. This appreciation is often cited as evidence of biophilia.

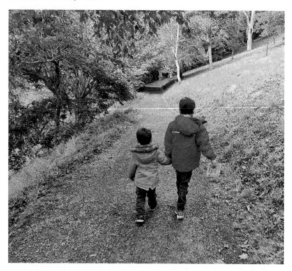

GLOSSARY

Biophilia
The passionate love of life and all that is alive.

EXERCISE 6.1   Nature in Language

Time for an activity. The symbolic use of nature in human language has been well established: for example, 'As dead as a dodo' and 'He/She was a social butterfly'. For a bit of fun, add the missing word to these sayings:

1 Busy as a _ _ _
2 _ _ _ headed
3 Let the _ _ _ out of the bag
4 Open a can of _ _ _ _ _
5 Going at a _ _ _ _ _ _ pace

6   Hold your _ _ _ _ _ _
7   The _ _ _ _ _ share
8   One trick _ _ _ _
9   _ _ _ _ _ _ _ _ in the room
10 Watching like a _ _ _ _
11 _ _ _ _ _ love
12 _ _ _ eat _ _ _
13 Let sleeping _ _ _ _ lie
14 Wild _ _ _ _ _ chase
15 The world is your _ _ _ _ _ _
16 _ _ _ _ in a china shop
17 A little _ _ _ _ told me
18 There are plenty more _ _ _ _ in the sea
19 Blind as a _ _ _
20 Eager _ _ _ _ _ _

The biophilia hypothesis has its roots in the evolutionary history of the human species when people had much closer contact with nature than most of us today living in concrete cities. This close connection with nature was required for survival against predators, poisonous plants and animals, and natural phenomena such as thunder and lightning. The technological advances of the nineteenth and twentieth centuries changed human interactions with nature for those of us living in more developed countries. However, nature is still an important need for many of us and vital in keeping us emotionally, psychologically, and physically healthy.

DID YOU KNOW?

Some of the evidence for our innate connection between humans and nature comes from studies of **biophobia** (the fear of nature), whereby measurable physiological responses are produced upon exposure to an object of fear, such as spiders or snakes. Our ancestors needed this close relationship with nature to 'read' the environment, using the sights and sounds around us as vital cues, particularly for the fight-or-flight response.

MENTAL HEALTH AND NATURE

In a recent survey conducted by the Mental Health Foundation, 73% of UK adults said that connecting with nature has been important for managing their mental health during the coronavirus pandemic. Other findings from this survey include the following (www.mentalhealth.org.uk/explore-mental-health/nature-mental-health):

- 70% of UK adults agreed that being close to nature improves their mood.
- 49% said that being close to nature helps them cope with stress.
- 34% of UK adults had connected more with nature during the pandemic.
- 45% of the UK population stated that parks helped them cope throughout the pandemic.

DID YOU KNOW?

A World Tree Hugging Championship is held in Halipuu Forest in Levi, Finland. This championship is meant to be fun; but tree hugging is said to create hormones similar to those released when we hug a loved one, such as oxytocin, which makes you feel calmer and happier. Oxytocin also causes a reduction in blood pressure, reduces the stress hormone norepinephrine, and produces a sense of relaxation.

You can take part remotely in the World Tree Hugging Championship (https://www.halipuu.com/treehuggingworldchampionships/): find your favourite tree, hug it, and take a picture. Then describe why you love this particular tree, and submit your entry. There are three categories: Speed Hugging, Dedication, and Freestyle Hugging!

MINDFUL MOMENT IN NATURE

Not long ago, my husband collected me from work with our two-year-old grandson in tow. It was such a lovely late afternoon that we decided to stop on the common for some playtime – blowing bubbles and kicking a football. My little grandson kicked the ball and ran after it as fast as his little legs could go – and then suddenly stopped abruptly and looked down at his feet in the grass. I immediately ran to him (thinking he had stepped in some dog poo or something)! But then I saw what he was looking at: a little daisy. He gazed at this daisy as if it was the most beautiful thing he had ever seen – a gem amongst gems. When I looked back to where I had run from (OK, hob-bled), I saw that I had stepped on a carpet of daisies and not even noticed. We picked the daisy he was looking at, and we touched it and smelled it whilst admiring its beauty. I did stop him from trying to eat it!

My grandson showed me mindfulness in action. We can all practice mindful moments in nature, paying attention to the present moment and spending time in green spaces to reduce our stress, anxiety, and depression whilst also combining this with gentle exercise. We will look at mindfulness in more detail in Chapter 13, but let's begin the process of combining mindfulness with nature in the next exercise.

EXERCISE 6.2   Mindfulness in Nature

1   Find a green space. When you get there, stop for a moment and take a deep breath.
2   Start exploring slowly. Try not to focus on getting somewhere in particular. Really focus on any movement you make. When walking, focus on which part of your foot touches the ground first, and feel the transfer of weight through your foot.
3   Notice the ground underneath you – is it grass or earth? Does it feel soft or hard? What colours can you see?
4   Think about the rest of your body. How are you holding your arms? Does the air on your face feel warm or cool?
5   Listen to the sounds around you. Can you hear bird songs or the wind rustling through the trees?
6   Look up at the sky and clouds. Does it look like rain? Look at the plants. Touch one, and focus on how it feels.
7   Smell the scents of nature around you. Are they floral or herby?
8   Enjoy the moment.

CONNECTING WITH NATURE

Not all of us have a connection with nature, which may have to be learned. Research has shown that this relationship comes through simple yet meaningful engagement with nature using five distinct types of activities that activate people's connection; see Table 6.2.

Table 6.2 The five pathways of connecting with nature.

1 Senses	Noticing and actively engaging with nature through the senses, such as listening to birdsong, smelling greenery/flowers, or watching the breeze in the trees
2 Emotion	Experiencing the joy and calm nature can bring, such as talking about and reflecting on your feelings about nature
3 Beauty	Taking the time to appreciate nature's beauty, such as exploring the beauty of nature through art or in music or words
4 Meaning	Celebrating how nature brings meaning to life, such as exploring how nature appears in songs, stories, poems, and art
5 Compassion	Taking actions that are good for nature, such as creating homes for nature and making ethical product choices

DID YOU KNOW?

Wildflowers are planted along roadside verges to improve biodiversity and cheer people up with the riot of colour. But this planting has also been found to have road safety implications, as it slows speeding drivers. So if you are ever travelling in the West Country in places such as between the villages of Tetbury and Malmsbury in the summer, have a look at the poppies and wildflowers along the verges along with the butterflies and bees.

SOUNDS OF NATURE

Research from the University of Exeter, England, has found that nature sounds benefit mental health.

EXERCISE 6.3   Nature Sounds

Go to a green space, and record the sounds of nature on your phone or other device. They may include bird songs, trees rustling in the wind, or, if you are lucky enough to live by the sea, the sounds of the waves. When you go to bed, replay these soothing sounds. If you wish, you can go on YouTube and obtain recordings of many nature sounds, such as rain against the window, thunderstorms, bird songs and more – but that would be cheating!

FOREST BATHING

Forest bathing is the Japanese practice of immersing yourself in nature in a mindful way. It is known in Japan as **shinrin-yoku** (*shinrin*, 'forest' and *yoku*, 'bathing'). Forest bathing began in the 1980s as an effective means to overcome the ill effects of a hectic life and work environment (Japan is known for being one of the most demanding work environments in the world). It is a useful tool to relax your mind, revitalise your body, and rediscover yourself.

DID YOU KNOW?

The **restoration theory** (Kaplan 1985) and **stress recovery theory** (Ulrich 1991) state that our recovery from stress starts within minutes of entering a green space. The physical body starts to calm down, blood pressure stabilises, stress hormones in our blood decrease, muscle tension relaxes – and the mental health benefits kick in. We start thinking more clearly, our feelings of vitality increase, and our mood lifts. It is thought that the time needed in nature for these benefits to manage our mental health is just 20 minutes per day.

Forest bathing has shown positive results across age groups, from children to the elderly, and is increasingly used by therapists and GPs alike and for employee recreation days. The benefits of forest bathing can be seen in Figure 6.1. (Like all the wellbeing strategies shown throughout this book, this stress-relieving method is not a replacement for medical advice or counselling for those who are seriously ill.)

Japan has over 70% forest coverage, so practising forest bathing is relatively easy. In the UK, we are not so lucky: only 13% of the total land area is covered by trees, woodlands, and forests (although it is hoped that this area will double by 2045 as a means of curbing the effects of climate change), so we may have to travel quite some distance to enjoy the benefits of forest bathing. But remember that those living in Tokyo and other city environments, as well as those of us in the UK, can practice this technique in green spaces and urban parks.

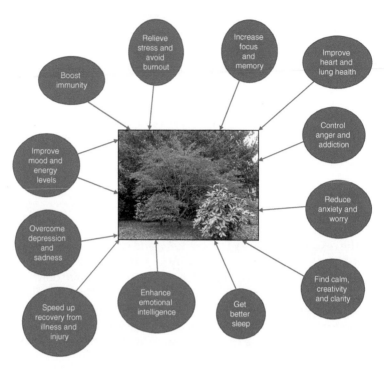

Figure 6.1 The benefits of forest bathing.

You can spend as little or as much time forest bathing as you wish, but the recommended time is at least two hours per week. The main principles of forest bathing are to go slow and to go in silence, using your senses to find things in nature that bring you peace and happiness. The stages of a 'forest mind' can be seen in Table 6.3.

You can evoke the sense of forest bathing by using meditation, as not everyone may feel safe in nature. Let's imagine a walk in the forest and enjoy Exercise 6.4.

Table 6.3 Stages of a forest mind.

Attention	**Beginners and young children start with simple activities focussing on objects in nature to hold our attention and slow us down.**
Awareness	**Once we are able to reach a calmer state of mind, we can grow our awareness of the nature around us.**
Answers	**Once our mind gets a well-deserved rest from all our mental chatter, it can apply itself with renewed energy.**

EXERCISE 6.4 The Forest Glade

Get comfortable, close your eyes, and let your imagination take you along a path in the forest.

Imagine you are standing at the edge of a field. It is a beautiful warm day.

Just a few yards away, you see a trail beginning at the tree line. You walk towards the path and enter the forest.

The light in the forest cascades down through the leaves in a soft spray.

The lower undergrowth is soft and green. Ferns and moss evoke a rich, herby smell.

The upper canopy of the trees covers you like a stained glass roof overhead, creating a soft, glowing, ambient light. The light is gentle and soothing.

You continue walking along the well-trodden path.

You notice the bark of the trees around you; some trunks have rough bark, some have smooth bark, some have light bark, and some have dark.

As you turn a corner, you see a small glade with a stream running through it. You continue towards it.

You hear the rippling water sounds, getting louder as you approach.

The swirling water looks crystal clear, and you can see rocks just under the surface.

You decide to sit on a large fallen tree. You slip off your shoes and dip your bare feet into the stream.

The water is very cold, but it instantly soothes your feet and refreshes you.

As the water massages your feet, you can hear the birds chirping overhead.

You smell the lush green pine trees around you. You also hear the gentle breeze fluttering through the leaves of the deciduous trees.

After you have rested a while, enjoying your surroundings, you decide it is time to leave this beautiful place. You put on your shoes.

You follow the path the way you came, back to the field.

Now open your eyes and come back to your awareness.

HOW TO GAIN THE BENEFITS OF NATURE

The previous exercise showed us that even though not all of us have the time, money, or ability to visit green or blue spaces, we can gain the benefits of nature through meditation. We can further our relationship with the natural world by writing a poem about our favourite nature spot, reflecting on a walk we once enjoyed, and looking at photographs we took during our foray into nature. In short, there are many ways we can get involved with nature, as we can see in Tables 6.4 and 6.5.

The benefits of nature can be gained intentionally. However, the benefits of nature can also be gained by incidental or indirect means:

Table 6.4 How to get involved with nature.

Make a bug hotel.	You can encourage nature and wildlife into your garden, if you are lucky enough to have one, by making a bug hotel or hedgehog house.
Grow some vegetables and herbs.	Vegetables like tomatoes and chilies and herbs such as chives, mint, basil, etc. are easy to grow in pots on a balcony or patio, or in a window box, and are good for you! There is nothing like the smell of fresh herbs.
Plant flowers.	Plant flowers such as sunflowers or lavender or anything that will attract the bees and butterflies, and sit and watch their beauty.
Take a dog for a walk.	Even if you don't have a dog, borrow one from a friend or neighbour and walk them, watching them run, sniff, and play.
Go on a nature walk.	Explore your local green spaces and woodlands. Take part in surveys such as the Royal Society for the Protection of Birds (RSPB) bird watch.
Go stargazing.	Stop and take time to look skywards and pinpoint constellations. Enjoy the Perseids meteorite shower in the UK between July 17 and August 24.
Notice the wildlife wherever you are.	Listen to the birdsong outside your window and the wildlife (squirrels, etc.) in your local park. If there is a pond nearby, feed the ducks with seed.

Table 6.5 How to bring the outside in.

Natural scents	Buy some scented candles, or spray natural fragrances, such as lavender or orange, around your house (see Chapter 9 on aromatherapy).
Indoor plants	Decorate your home with green plants. You can use artificial plants to evoke the feeling of nature if you don't have green fingers.
Arts and craft	On your forays into nature, collect natural materials like driftwood, sea glass, shells, pebbles, feathers, etc., and make something with them.
Interior design	Buy floral duvets and cushions with scenes of nature on them to bring nature to your home.
Sounds from the natural world	Go on YouTube to access natural sounds, such as waves, birdsong, rain falling, thunder, etc. Close your eyes and relax to these sounds.
Nature programmes	Another way of bringing nature to you, especially if you live in the middle of a city, is to watch a nature documentary. Research has suggested that watching a nature programme can have the same benefits as doing meditation.

Intentional – Interacting with nature by going to green or blue spaces or spending time in your garden

Incidental – Carrying out our daily activities like driving to work or walking to the shops

Indirect – When we are not present in nature, watching a nature programme or looking out a window (Table 6.5)

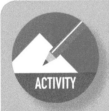

Chapter 6 Activity

Depending on the season, enjoy these nature activities:

Winter – Make a snowperson or go for a ride on a sledge.

Autumn – Go for a walk in some woodlands – crunching the leaves beneath your feet.

Summer – Pick some flowers, press the petals, and make bookmarks by laminating them.

Spring – Buy a couple of pots, and grow some mint and other herbs. Enjoy eating them when ready.

KEY POINTS

- The health benefits of nature
- The biophilia hypothesis
- Mental health and nature
- Mindful moments in nature
- Connecting with nature
- Sounds of nature
- Forest bathing (shinrin-yoku)
- How to gain the benefits of nature

WEB RESOURCES

- **Health benefits of nature:** https://www.bupa.co.uk/ newsroom/ourviews/nature-wellbeing
- *The Lancet*: https://www.thelancet.com/pdfs/journals/ lancet/p1150140-6736(08)61689-x.pdf
- **Nature and mental health:** https://www.mentalhealth.org. uk/explore-mental-health/nature-mental-health
- **National Park Service USA:** https://www.nps.gov/articles/ naturesbenefits.htm#
- **The biophilia hypothesis:** https://www.britannica.com/ science/biophilia-hypothesis
- **The benefits of nature sounds:** www.bbc.co.uk/news/ uk-england-devon-60840759
- **Restoration theory (Kaplan 1985):** https:// positivepsychology.com/attention-restoration-theory
- **Stress recovery theory (Ulrich 1991):** https://www. sageglass.com/en/visionary-insights/stress-reduction-theory
- **Tree Hugging World Championships:** https://www. halipuu.com/treehuggingworldchampionships/

Chapter 7

• • • • • • • • • • • • • • • • • • • •

NUTRITION, HYDRATION, AND EXERCISE

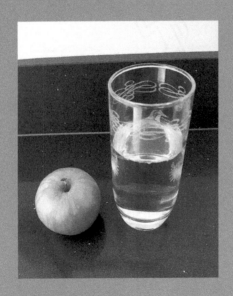

Wellbeing Strategies for Nurses, First Edition. Claire Boyd.
© 2023 John Wiley & Sons Ltd. Published 2023 by John Wiley & Sons Ltd.

LEARNING OUTCOMES

By the end of this chapter, you will have an understanding of the importance of a balanced diet, good hydration, and physical activity for our wellbeing. You will also know how to achieve a balanced diet and good hydration; what counts as moderate, vigorous, and very rigorous activity; and how diet, hydration, and exercise can affect our moods.

During this chapter, we will look at how stress can be helped by eating well, keeping hydrated, and exercising – but not all at the same time! Unfortunately, during busy shifts at the hospital, it is often a case of our feet not touching the ground from the time we start work to the time we go home (often on our knees).

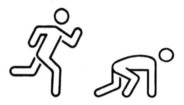

To start with, during the fight-or-flight stress response, our body prepares for a perceived attack and is not concerned with digestion, leaving any food in our guts un-metabolized and the digestive system very sluggish. This can:

- Cause the oesophagus to go into spasm
- Increase the acid in our stomachs, which may result in indigestion
- Make us feel nauseous
- Give us diarrhoea or constipation

THE IMPORTANCE OF GOOD NUTRITION FOR OUR WELLBEING

Good health often starts with good nutrition, which involves eating a balanced diet. Unfortunately, studies have found that stress can affect our food preferences: physical or emotional stress increases the intake of foods high in fat, sugar, or both – which you may have heard referred to 'comfort foods'. This is when we grab a chocolate or biscuit instead of a celery stick!

DID YOU KNOW?

Stress wears down the immune system, which is why we often fall ill during stressful times in our lives.

We all need a 'balanced diet' – but what exactly does that mean? A **balanced diet** gives the body the nutrients it needs to function correctly. Most of the calories should come from:

- Fresh fruits
- Fresh vegetables
- Whole grains
- Legumes
- Nuts
- Lean proteins

Calories are the amount of energy stored in food, which the body uses to function (breathing, walking, thinking, etc.). On average, an adult requires about 2000 calories every day to maintain their weight, but this depends on factors such as age, gender, and physical activity level; for example, a female centenarian does not require the same calories as a male 25-year-old marathon runner. Note that a centenarian (a person 100+ years old) is not the same as a centurion (a Roman soldier)! Table 7.1 shows the guidelines for calorie intake.

Where we get these calories is another important factor, as foods with high calorific content may have very little nutritional benefit – these are known as **empty calories**. Examples of foods that provide empty calories include:

- Cakes, biscuits, and doughnuts
- Processed meats
- Energy drinks and soft drinks
- Fruit drinks with added sugar
- Ice cream
- Crisps and chips
- Pizza

Table 7.1 Suggested guidelines for calorie intake.

Children	2–8 years old	1000–14 000
Males	9–13 years old	1600–2600
Active females	14–30 years old	2400
Sedentary females	14–30 years old	1800–2000
Active males	14–30 years old	2800–3200
Sedentary males	14–30 years	2000–2600
Active people	30 years and over	2000–3000
Sedentary people	30 years and over	1600–2400

In other words, all the nice stuff! We need to limit our consumption of empty calories and try to get our calories from foods that are rich in other nutrients to achieve a balanced diet.

DID YOU KNOW?

It is estimated that more than 21 million adults in the UK will be obese by the year 2040, which equates to 36% of the adult population. If the trends continue, the number of people in the UK who are obese will overtake the number who are a healthy weight.

Without a balanced diet, our bodies do not get the nutrients the body requires to work effectively, making us more prone to disease, infection, fatigue, and low performance.

What to Eat for a Balanced Diet

A Balanced diet usually includes:

- Vitamins, minerals, and antioxidants
- Carbohydrates
- Protein
- Healthy fats

A balanced diet also includes a variety of foods from the following groups:

- Fruits
- Vegetables
- Grains
- Dairy
- Protein foods (such as meat, eggs, fish, beans, nuts, and legumes)

For those following a plant-based diet, proteins can be obtained from:

- Lentils
- Beans
- Peas
- Almonds
- Sunflower seeds
- Walnuts
- Tofu
- Tempeh (soy-based alternative to meat)

DID YOU KNOW?

If you follow a vegan diet, there are many dairy-free milks and other dairy alternatives made from soy, almonds, oats, coconut, cashews, hazelnut, flax seeds, etc.

When we are stressed, we may reach for processed and empty-calorie foods because they are quick, but this will affect our health and often make the situation worse. It is important that we all look after ourselves, including eating a healthy diet, which begins with breakfast. Have a go at making some overnight oats!

EXERCISE 7.1   Overnight Oats

1   Combine dry oats with milk or yoghurt – jumbo oats will add more texture than normal porridge oats.
2   Add some coarsely grated apple or pear to the mixture.
3   Pour into a large jam jar (clean and empty, of course).
4   Leave overnight in the fridge.
5   The next day the oats will be softened. Stir.
6   Customize with seasonal fruit/berries or seeds.
7   Drizzle with honey, if you wish.

VITAMINS AND MINERALS

It is essential that we get 'essential' vitamins and minerals from our diet – hence they are called 'essential'! An important compound in the body is sodium chloride, which is used to:

- Absorb and transport nutrients around the body
- Help maintain blood pressure
- Maintain the right balance of fluids in the body
- Transmit nerve signals
- Contract and relax muscles

Table 7.2 shows some other essential vitamins and minerals required by the body.

When we don't get enough of certain vitamins and minerals, our mental and physical health is affected. Table 7.3 shows how different vitamin/mineral deficiencies can affect our mood.

A healthy balanced diet should provide you with all the nutrients your body requires.

Happy Foods

Certain foods have been shown to reduce anxiety, but this does not mean eating these 'happy foods' will transform your mood instantly:

- Mackerel
- Marmite (brewer's yeast)
- Chilies
- Oats

Table 7.2 Some of the essential vitamins and minerals.

Vitamin A	Promotes good eyesight, growth, and healthy skin and muscle
Vitamin B complex (B1, B2, B9, B12, folic acid)	Niacin helps increase energy, and folic acid is important in pregnancy.
Vitamin C	Helps in the absorption of calcium and iron and in wound healing
Vitamin D	Helps in the absorption of calcium for healthy teeth and bones
Vitamin E	Helps to protect cells from damage
Vitamin K	Blood coagulation
Magnesium	Bones, muscles, and nerves
Potassium	Heart and nerve cells
Iodine	Thyroid
Iron	Lungs, blood
Zinc	Digestion, metabolism
Selenium	Inflammation, heart
Chromium	Metabolism, blood sugar

Table 7.3 Vitamin/mineral deficiencies and mood.

Iron	A lack of iron can make us feel weak, tired, and lethargic.
B vitamins	A lack of B1, B3, and B12 can make us feel tired, irritable, and low in mood.
Folate	A lack of folate can make us feel depressed.
Selenium	A lack of selenium may increase the chance of feeling depressed and other negative mood states.

- Brazil nuts
- Lettuce
- Leafy green vegetables

Studies have also found other mood boosters, which can be seen in Table 7.4.

Table 7.4 'Happy foods'.

Avocado	This fruit is rich in monounsaturated fats. According to a 2020 study, eating more fats like the ones in avocado is associated with a lower anxiety score in women. Avocados are also high in B vitamins, which are associated with lower stress levels and may help improve mood.
Dark chocolate	Research in 2020 found that cocoa helps to improve brain performance in young adults, whilst a study in 2019 also found that eating dark chocolate (with a high cocoa content) was associated with a lower risk of depressive symptoms.
Coffee	A 2016 review found caffeine intake is associated with lower levels of depression and anxiety. Coffee also contains antioxidants, which are linked to lowering inflammation.
Black beans	Magnesium deficiency is linked to anxiety and low energy levels. Black beans are rich in magnesium – which helps boost serotonin levels – and also contain vital nutrients such as iron, copper, fibre, zinc, and potassium.
Coconut	Coconuts contain medium-chain triglycerides (fatty acids), and a study in 2018 found that these fatty acids may help reduce anxiety.
Eggs	Egg yolks are high in choline – which helps regulate mood – and omega-3s, zinc, B vitamins, iodine, and protein.
Red peppers	If you are low on iron and feel tired, eating raw red pepper with iron-rich foods can help with your energy levels and give you an injection of mood-boosting vitamin C.
Red wine	Wine contains high amounts of resveratrol, which has been linked to depression relief, according to a 2013 study. This study looked at the occasional glass of red wine in reducing depression risk.
Seaweed	Seaweed contains iodine, which is essential for healthy thyroid production, which in turn has an impact on energy levels and mood.
Salmon	Salmon contains omega-3s, which may boost your mood. Studies in 2013 and 2016 found a strong relationship between higher omega-3 intake and lower rates of depression.
Beetroot	Beetroot contains high levels of folate, and a study in 2017 found that people without depression had higher folate levels than those with.

Table 7.4 (*Continued*)

Honey	Honey contains healthy compounds like kaempferol and quercetin that may keep depressive symptoms at bay.
Whole-grain bread	Complex carbohydrates like whole-grain bread help settle chemical messengers without crashing your system later.
Bananas	Bananas contain serotonin, the happy hormone.
Blueberries	Blueberries are a good source of polyphenols and antioxidants. All dark berries contain vitamin C, which a 2018 study found was associated with elevated mood in male students.
Almonds	Almonds are full of magnesium, a mineral that helps manage cortisol levels.
Oranges	Oranges and other citrus fruits contain vitamin C, which can lower blood pressure.

EXERCISE 7.2   Treat Yourself

This is probably the nicest exercise in the book. Treat yourself to a bar of dark chocolate – enjoy!

THE IMPORTANCE OF GOOD HYDRATION FOR WELLBEING

Good hydration is critical for health and wellbeing, as almost every mechanism in our bodies relies on adequate water intake. A study found that hydration plays an important part in our mental health, too – drinking the least water doubled the risk of depression and anxiety. For a body already experiencing stress, this is compounding the situation.

When we are in a state of dehydration, our cognitive performance is affected. Studies have shown that being dehydrated by just 2% impairs things like memory and focusing on daily tasks. Reducing water intake can also lower your mood, as dehydration creates a stressor on the body – which impacts mood-boosting hormones such as serotonin and increases stress hormones. Another study found that those who reduced their water intake increased their thirst, which decreased positive emotions such as calmness and feeling content. Those who drank less water and increased their intake reported improved fatigue and an improvement in their mood when waking up at the start of the day.

Studies have also shown that those experiencing sleep problems, perhaps due to anxiety and stress, and therefore sleeping for shorter periods each night are more likely to be dehydrated. This can create a cycle of not sleeping and reaching for coffee or other energy drinks when we are low on energy. Caffeine is a diuretic, which increases our need to urinate, meaning we lose more fluids. We should therefore increase our fluid intake to compensate for this. Alcohol also works in a similar way to caffeine.

STUDENT TIP

This does not mean we can't drink caffeine or alcohol ever again, just that we need to drink more water to balance things out.

DEHYDRATION

To avoid dehydration, we should all know how much water we drink. It is easy to lose track, especially during a busy shift. Tracker bottles are useful for this, including those with graduated lines showing how much water you should have drunk by certain times of the day; then you can drink more if you are falling behind.

DID YOU KNOW?

Jelly drops: These are drops containing 95% water with added electrolytes. They are sugar-free, gluten-free, and vegan, with natural flavourings. Each sweet contains 12.5 mL water. They are good for patients and service users who are not drinking enough, as a way to increase hydration, and were developed by a team of designers, engineers, and food scientists. Some nurses have also taken to using them as a quick fix between having proper drinks.

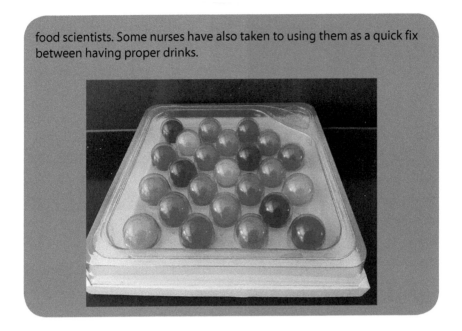

Many of us are unaware when we are dehydrated, so it is important to learn to read the signs and act as needed. Signs of dehydration include:

- Dark urine
- Less urination
- Thirst
- Dry mouth
- Constipation
- Fatigue
- Headache
- Lightheadedness
- Muscle cramps
- Rapid heartbeat
- Low blood pressure
- Dry lips and cracked mouth

In severe cases, signs can include:

- Delirium
- Unconsciousness

HIGH-WATER-CONTENT FRUITS AND VEGETABLES

You can also get extra water into your body by ingesting foods with high water content. Table 7.5 shows some fruits and vegetables that have high water content.

Table 7.5 High-water-content fruits and vegetables.

Food	Water percentage
Watermelon	92%
Strawberries	92%
Cantaloupe	90%
Pineapple	87%
Cucumber	96%
Blueberries	85%
Lettuce	96%
Celery	95%
Tomato	94%
Grapefruit	91%
Pear	92%
Apple	92%
Grapes	81%
Spinach	92%
Cabbage	93%
Radishes	95%
Peach	88%
Apricot	86%
Orange	87%
Bell peppers	92%
Cranberries	87%
Cauliflower	92%
Broccoli	91%
Raspberries	87%

You can also get more fluids into the body from foods such as ice cream, jelly, soup, ice lollies, etc. The next exercise shows how to make fruit ice lollies.

EXERCISE 7.3   Fruit Ice Lollies

You will need:

- 400g strawberries, hulled and roughly chopped
- 150g natural yoghurt
- 30g caster sugar (or 2 tablespoons honey)

1   Blitz the strawberries to a puree.
2   Add the yoghurt, and blitz again to combine.
3   Taste for sweetness, and add sugar or honey.
4   Divide the mixture evenly between six ice-lolly moulds (fill to the brim).
5   Insert wooden sticks, and freeze for four hours or until set.

These ice lollies will keep up to one month in the freezer.

Caffeine

We have already seen that coffee can be considered a 'happy food', but consuming too much caffeine may worsen feelings of anxiety and disrupt sleep.

Caffeine is a chemical found in coffee, tea, chocolate, and energy drinks and is known to stimulate the central nervous system. We all have different thresholds for how much caffeine we can tolerate, but it is recommended to keep caffeine intake to under 400 mg per day – which equates to four or five cups (900–1200 mg) of coffee.

EXERCISE 7.4   Making Changes

If your caffeine intake is above the recommended daily amount, replace one of your usual drinks with either herbal tea or a plain glass of water.

THE IMPORTANCE OF EXERCISE FOR WELLBEING

Technology may be a good thing because it makes our lives easier, but it has meant that many people are less active nowadays, which is obviously a bad thing. Research has shown that many adults spend more than seven hours a day sitting down: at work, on transport, and during their leisure time. Sedentary lifestyles include such behaviours as watching television; using a computer; using the car for short journeys; and sitting down to read, talk, or listen to music. According to the Department of Health, this inactivity is a 'silent killer'. Those who do regular physical activity have a lower risk of:

- Coronary heart disease and stroke
- Type 2 diabetes
- Bowel cancer
- Breast cancer in women
- Early death
- Osteoarthritis
- Hip fracture
- Falls
- Depression
- Dementia

The National Health Service has developed guidelines for adults aged 19–64, showing the types of physical exercises we should aim to achieve every day. However, exercising just once or twice a week can reduce the risk of heart disease or stroke.

Adults should aim to:

- Do strengthening activities that work on all the major muscle groups (legs, hips, back, abdomen, chest, shoulders, and arms) at least two days a week.
- Do at least 150 minutes of moderate-intensity activity a week or 75 minutes of vigorous-intensity activity a week.
- Spread exercise evenly over four to five days a week, or every day.
- Reduce time spent sitting or lying down, and break up long periods of not moving with some activity.

It is suggested that you can achieve the weekly activity target by:

- Doing several short sessions of very vigorous intensity activity
- Doing a mix of moderate-intensity, vigorous-intensity, and very-vigorous-intensity activity

What counts as moderate aerobic activity, vigorous activity, and very vigorous activity? Table 7.6 explains with examples.

High-Intensity Training (HIT)

We saw that high-intensity training (HIT) is part of a very rigorous exercise routine, but what exactly is it? HIT involves short bursts of intense exercise with short recovery

Table 7.6 Moderate aerobic, vigorous, and very vigorous activity.

Moderate aerobic activity	Vigorous activity	Very vigorous activity
This type of activity will raise your heart rate and make you breathe faster and feel warmer. One way of telling whether you have achieved a moderate intensity level is that you can still talk but not sing! Examples of this type of activity are:	This type of activity makes you breathe hard and fast. One way of telling whether you have achieved a vigorous level is that you cannot say more than a few words without pausing for breath. Examples of this type of activity are:	Very vigorous activities are exercises performed in short bursts of maximum effort broken up with rest. This type of exercise is also known as high-intensity training (HIT) or high-intensity interval training (HIIT). Examples of this type of activity are:
<ul><li>Brisk walking</li><li>Water aerobics</li><li>Riding a bike</li><li>Dancing</li><li>Doubles tennis</li><li>Pushing a lawn mower</li><li>Hiking</li><li>Rollerblading</li></ul>	<ul><li>Running</li><li>Swimming</li><li>Riding a bike fast on hills</li><li>Walking up the stairs</li><li>Sports, e.g. football, rugby, netball, hockey</li><li>Skipping</li><li>Aerobics</li><li>Gymnastics</li><li>Martial arts</li></ul>	<ul><li>Lifting heavy weights</li><li>Circuit training</li><li>Sprinting up hills</li><li>Interval running</li><li>Running up stairs</li><li>Spinning classes</li></ul>

breaks in between. There are various forms of HIT, but an example of this type of exercise is as follows, using an exercise bike:

1   Warm up for a couple of minutes with some gentle cycling. Then cycle as fast as you possibly can for 20 seconds.
2   Cycle gently again for a couple of minutes whilst you catch your breath, and then do another 20 seconds flat out.
3   For the final time, cycle gently for 2 minutes to catch your breath, followed by a third period of 20 seconds flat out.
4   Finished!

Research shows that doing 10 one-minute sprints on a stationary exercise bike with about one minute of rest in between, three times a week, is as good for improving muscle as many hours of less strenuous conventional long-term biking.

Three-Minute Exercise Formula for a Longer Life

Scientists from Glasgow Caledonian University (Scotland) found that performing three minutes of moderate exercise for each hour of the day you spend sitting down could cut your chance of early death by 30%. Table 7.7 shows what we should be doing every hour/on the hour.

STUDENT TIP

I suggest you might want to go to the toilet to empty your bladder before attempting jumping jacks – just saying!

DID YOU KNOW?

Family doctors will now prescribe walking and cycling in a national push to boost both mental and physical health. Pilot studies will run until 2025 in 11 local authorities in England.

Table 7.7 Three-minute exercise routine.

Jumping jacks × 50 seconds Rest for 10 seconds.	1	Stand upright with your legs together, arms at your sides.
	2	Bend your knees slightly, and jump in the air.
	3	As you jump, spread your legs to about shoulder-width apart. Stretch your arms out and over your head.
	4	Jump back to your starting position.
	5	Repeat.
Press-ups × 50 seconds Rest for 10 seconds.	1	Lie on the floor, face down.
	2	Press your toes against the floor and place your hands flat on the ground, shoulder-width apart, fingers extended forward.
	3	Push yourself up so your arms are nearly extended and your torso and legs are off the floor. This is your starting position.
	4	Inhaling, bend your arms to lower your body and touch your chest nearly to the floor.
	5	Exhaling, contract your chest as you push off the ground and return to the starting position.
	6	Pause for a moment and then repeat.
Bodyweight squats × 50 seconds Rest for 10 seconds.	1	Stand straight with your feet hip-width apart, toes facing forward.
	2	Drive your hips back, bending at the knees and ankles. Press your knees slightly open as you bend down. Sit into a squat position while still keeping your heels and toes on the ground, chest up and shoulders back (work to reach parallel = knees bent to a 90° angle).
	3	Press into your heels and straighten your legs, pressing through your knees to return to the standing position.
	4	Pause for a moment and then repeat.

Exercise Can Make you Happier

Exercise is good not only for our physical body but also for our mental wellbeing. When we are stressed, exercise can help lift our mood. Table 7.8 shows 17 ways in which exercise can make us happier. Note: Ribbons are optional!

Table 7.8 17 ways exercise may make you happier.

Helps reduce anxiety	Studies show that just 5 minutes of exercise can brighten our mood.
Boosts brain power	Exercise can increase concentration levels by improving blood flow to the brain.
Strengthens the immune system	Exercise can raise our body temperature and flush bacteria from the body.
Helps with sleep	Better sleep = better mood, memory, and overall health.
Helps develop self-discipline	Studies show people with good self-discipline are happier.
Improves body-image perception	Exercise may improve the way you feel about yourself.
Better posture	Strong muscles encourage strong posture.
Eases joint pain	When muscles are strong, this takes the pressure off our joints.
Gives you a 'runner's high'	Exercise releases endorphins.
Gives you energy	With exercise, the body is filled with fresh oxygenated blood when the heart pumps faster.
Sharpens your memory	Studies show that people who exercise are better at difficult tasks involving the memory.
May get you outdoors	Studies show that people who spend a little time outdoors have less stress.
Helps you meet new people	Friends are good for our mental health, and we may meet people in parks, gyms, etc.
Helps you lose weight	Exercise leads to better physical health.
Lowers your risk of injury	Exercise trains the muscles how to move properly.
Brightens the skin	Sweating removes toxins from the body and increases blood flow.
Helps fight insulin resistance	When you exercise, you burn sugar in your muscles (while your body recovers, it takes sugar from your bloodstream).

The Benefits of a Brisk Walk and Exercise

Leicester University researchers looked at genetic data on 400 000 adults from the UK Biobank with an average age of 57 and recorded their walking pace. The researchers found that faster walkers had longer telomeres regardless of how much they exercised. **Telomeres** are the 'caps' at the end of chromosomes that protect them and are regarded as strong markers for biological age. The difference in telomere length between the fastest and slowest walkers in the study was found to be equivalent to 16 more years of life.

EXERCISE 7.5 Go Walking

Put on your trainers and go for a brisk walk around your neighbourhood.

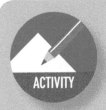

Chapter 7 Activity

You have read this chapter, but how many of you actually did the three-minute exercise routine? Go on, get up a sweat, and let's do these exercises:

* Jumping jacks × 50 seconds (rest for 10 seconds)
* Press-ups × 50 seconds (rest for 10 seconds)
* Bodyweight squats × 50 seconds (rest for 10 seconds)

KEY POINTS

* The importance of good nutrition for wellbeing
* What to eat for a balanced diet
* Vitamins and minerals

- Happy foods
- The importance of good hydration for wellbeing
- Dehydration
- High-water-content fruit and vegetables
- The importance of exercise for wellbeing
- High-intensity training (HIT)
- Three-minute exercise formula for a longer life
- Exercise can make you happier
- The benefits of a brisk walk and exercise

WEB RESOURCES

- **Exercise makes us happy:** https://relaxlikeaboss.com/relaxation-techniques
- **Three-minute exercise:** https://mensfitness.co.uk/fitness/3-minute-exercise-formula-for-longer-life, https://www.weforum.org/agenda/2021/06/three-minutes-exercise-longer-life
- **Walking for health:** http://www.nhs.uk/live-well/exercise/running-and-aerobic-exercises/walking-for-health
- **Exercise guidelines:** http://www.nhs.uk/live-well/exercise/exercise-guidelines
- **Live well:** http://www.nhs.uk/live-well
- **Department of Health and Social Care physical activity guidelines:** http://www.gov.uk/government/publications/physical-activity-guidelines-infographics
- **Hydration:** https://www.nhsinform.scot/campaigns/hydration
- **Balanced diet:** https://www.toppr.com/guides/science/components-of-foods/balanced-diet/, https://www.livescience.com/why-a-balanced-diet-is-important

Chapter 8

· · · · · · · · · · · · · · · · · · · ·

COLOUR THERAPY

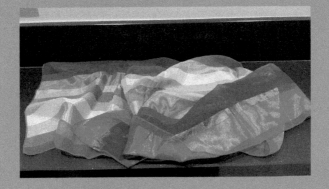

LEARNING OUTCOMES

By the end of this chapter, you will have an understanding of the colour spectrum, wavelengths, and how we see colours. You will also know how colours are used in everyday language and in colour therapy, the environment, clothing, and foods for their health benefits.

Colour therapy and healing (also known as **chromotherapy** or **light therapy**) is a form of holistic healing that uses the visible spectrum of light and colour to affect a person's mood and physical or mental health. The belief is that cells and organs vibrate at certain frequencies, and colour therapists believe that colour can be used to correct vibrational imbalances in the body to create balance, good health, and wellbeing. The colour is absorbed into the body through the eyes and skin, much like a transdermal patch.

The main idea behind colour therapy is that different colours evoke different responses in people. Some colours are considered to be more stimulating and energising, whilst others are more soothing and calming. Based on this idea, it is thought that colour exposure can impact our overall mood, motivation, sleep, outlook, etc.

Certain aspects of chromotherapy have undergone more robust research, such as environmental and psychology studies in areas such as marketing and advertising.

DID YOU KNOW?

Studies have shown that looking at the colour red increased the heart rate and caused the BP to rise due to the colour's stimulating effect.

Looking at the calming colour blue resulted in a slower heart rate and lower BP.

Yellow, orange, and red in the classroom can increase learning and IQ.

Other claims can be said to be more dubious: When I undertook a colour therapy course, we were told such things as to wear an indigo cotton or silk scarf around the head for headaches and a red one around the neck for a sore throat!

All I can say is that no evidence was supplied regarding this 'treatment' when requested. It is evident that a lot more research needs to be conducted into the effectiveness of this therapy!

CHROMOTHERAPY TREATMENT

The instrument used to deliver colour treatment consists of two glass-fronted boxes placed side by side on a table or stand. Inside each box is a lamp with slots for stained glass filters to be inserted, with alternating colours. The therapy involves shining single or mixed colours on the whole body or particular areas of the body.

Some colour therapists have expanded the therapy to use colour crystals by placing them on the corresponding chakra area. Some also use swatches of coloured silk or aura-soma (balancing bottles of coloured liquid). Some therapists prefer to concentrate on the colours of the environment or our clothing to see how these may affect our emotions and wellbeing.

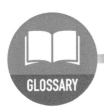

GLOSSARY

Chakras

These are believed to be energy centres in the body that correspond to specific nerve bundles and internal organs. Seven major chakras run along from base of the spine up to the crown of the head. To function effectively, the chakras must stay open and balanced. If they are blocked, physical or emotional symptoms may manifest, related to a particular chakra. Each chakra point is represented by a colour:

- Base of coccyx – Red
- Lower abdomen – Orange
- Solar plexus – Yellow
- Heart – Green
- Throat – Blue
- Forehead – Violet/Indigo
- Crown – Magenta or white

TOOLS USED IN COLOUR THERAPY

As stated earlier, colour therapists use a variety of tools. Following is a full list of ways this treatment can be applied:

- Stained-glass filters
- Coloured crystals (often placed on chakra points)
- Silk scarves
- Coloured water/oils (known as **auras**)
- Coloured card swatches
- Clothing
- Environment (choosing colours for rooms)
- Food (such as the **rainbow diet**)
- Visualisation (see Chapter 14)
- Colour breathing (meditation)

HISTORY OF COLOUR THERAPY

Many ancient civilisations, such as the Egyptians, Greeks, and Chinese, used the perceived healing properties of colour to restore health and vitality in individuals. Today, colour therapists believe that different colours can treat physical and mental health and improve mind, body, and spirit. This is because colour can evoke moods and feelings in individuals; for example, some people feel happy when wearing their favourite colour.

Colours of the Spectrum

Isaac Newton discovered that when light entered a prism, the light was refracted or deflected into the colours of the spectrum. Each colour had a different angle of refraction, making it visible to the human eye. When he turned the prism down, the colours combined to form white light again.

Newton also concluded that each light or colour consisted of waves and that each colour has a different wavelength and vibrates at a different frequency, from high to low energy. Table 8.1 shows the wavelengths of the colours in the spectrum.

Table 8.1 Colour spectrum wavelengths.

High energy	Colour	Wavelength
	Violet	380 nm
	Indigo	445 nm
	Blue	450 nm
	Green	495 nm
	Yellow	570 nm
	Orange	590 nm
Low energy	Red	620 nm

DID YOU KNOW?

Nm = nanometre and equates to a thousand-millionth of a metre.

EXERCISE 8.1 Make a Newton Illusion Wheel

Trace around an old CD on a thin white card, and cut out the circle. Then divide the circle into sections, and colour each section using the colours red, orange, yellow, green, blue, violet. Snip out a small hole in the middle of the circle, and thread some string or wool through the hole. Start spinning! You will see all the colours disappear and see white only.

The spectrum consists of seven colours – mainly violet, indigo, blue, green, yellow, orange, and red – all of which appear as white (or off-white or grey) when the wheel spins very fast.

COLOUR IDIOMS

Colour is all around us: in nature, our home décor, the clothes we wear, and the food we eat. Moods have also long been associated with colours, and we often use colour words to express our emotions, such as 'feeling blue', meaning feeling down in the dumps.

EXERCISE 8.2   Idiom Quiz

For a bit of fun, how many of these idioms have you heard of? Do you know their meaning?

	Idiom	Meaning
1	A red rag to a bull	
2	As brown as a berry	
3	As white as a sheet/ghost	
4	Black sheep of the family	
5	Browned off	
6	Caught red-handed	
7	Every cloud has a silver lining	
8	In the pink	
9	Once in a blue moon	
10	Paint the town red	
11	Purple patch	
12	Red herring	
13	Red letter day	
14	Red tape	
15	The grass is always greener on the other side of the fence	
16	Tickled pink	
17	Roll out the red carpet	
18	Green thumb	
19	Got the green light	
20	Green with envy	
21	Red in the face	
22	It was black and white	
23	Golden opportunity	
24	Grey area	
25	Rose-coloured glasses	
26	White elephant	

Idiom	Meaning
27 A bolt from the blue	
28 The pot calling the kettle black	
29 Blueblood	
30 White lie	

HOW WE SEE COLOURS

Most of us see colour due to millions of **rods** and **cones**: light-receptive sensors in the retinas of our eyes. The rods are sensitive to low light, and the cones are sensitive to colour and require a greater light intensity. The optic nerve receives the message, which is then passed on to the brain.

Our eyes can only detect three colours: red, green, and blue. By combining these, we can perceive many different colours. For example, by mixing red and green light, we can see yellow; and by mixing red and blue, we can see violet.

Objects absorb and reflect light differently: a red apple reflects red light, and all the other colours of the spectrum are absorbed and so are not seen by our eyes. Black does not reflect any light at all, whereas with white, all the colours are reflected.

Sunlight is a mixture of all the colours of light, which combine to form brilliant white light. Some surfaces reflect all of this light, while others only absorb some of the colours.

DID YOU KNOW?

One in 12 men and 1 in 200 women cannot distinguish between certain colours, mainly shades of red, yellow, and green. This is called **colour vision deficiency** or colour blindness.

THE IMPORTANCE OF COLOUR

In the summer, when the sun is shining, we tend to spend more time outdoors. Being in the sunlight helps to create strong, healthy bones. This is because we absorb ultraviolet light through our eyes, which enables the body to produce vitamin D, essential for the metabolisation of calcium. We know that ultraviolet light cannot pass through glass, so wearing glasses or sunglasses or even contact lenses can inhibit its absorption.

When the days become shorter and autumn arrives, our exposure to sunlight is diminished. A condition resulting from this light deprivation is seasonal affective disorder (SAD). The effects of SAD can be depression, a desire to sleep, lethargy, and often an increased craving for carbohydrates. Treatment for SAD may include cognitive behaviour therapy, antidepressants, and/or light therapy to treat the person's mood.

Light therapy involves sitting by a special lamp called a **light box** for around 30 minutes to an hour each day, usually in the morning. These boxes produce a very bright light. The intensity of the light is measured in lux; the higher the lux, the brighter the light. Figure 8.1 shows a typical light box.

The light box's light simulates the sunlight that is missing during the winter months. It is thought that the light may improve SAD by encouraging the brain to reduce the production of melatonin (a hormone that makes you feel sleepy) and increases the production of serotonin (a hormone that affects your mood).

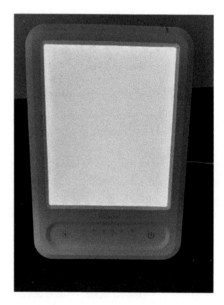

Figure 8.1 Light box.

SCIENCE OF COLOUR THERAPY

Colour Therapy has its foundations in colour energy, based on the theory that the vibrations of colour waves directly affect the cells and organs of the body. Each colour has a specific wavelength and frequency with its own vibration. Albert Einstein proved that the spectrum of colours is composed of small packets of energy called **photons**. The longer the wavelength, the more spaced out the photons. Blue, indigo, and violet have compacted photons with short wavelengths. These wavelengths contain the most energy. The colours at the other end of the spectrum have longer wavelengths with less energy.

COMMON COLOURS USED DURING COLOUR THERAPY

Interior designers and psychologists claim that the colour of a room can affect individuals using these rooms, as colours are thought to treat various conditions.

DID YOU KNOW?

In 1903, the *Boston Globe* printed an article called 'Colours That Will Drive the Brain to Madness'. The story included such statements as 'purple is the most dangerous colour there is', and 'deep purple will kill you eventually'!

Here is a list of the most common colours used during colour therapy and their perceived attributes.

Colour	Attributes
Red	Used to energise or invigorate: especially good when feeling tired or lacklustre.
Blue	Used to treat depression or pain. Darker shades are thought to have sedative properties and to be useful for people who experience insomnia or other sleeping disorders.
Green	The colour of nature, used to relieve stress and relax individuals.
Yellow	Used to improve the mood, helping elevate happiness and optimism.
Orange	Used to elicit happy emotions from people. This warm colour is also thought to stimulate appetite and mental activity.

Other colours that colour therapists may choose to work with include these:

Turquoise	Made up of blue and green. Used to create emotional balance and stability.
Violet	Made up of blue and red, with an emphasis on red. Used to aid sleep and sleep disorders and stress.
Magenta	Made up of red and violet. Used to assist when someone feels anger and frustration or is worried or despondent, as an aid to 'letting go'.
Indigo	Made up of red and blue, with an emphasis on blue. Used to assist in creating a balanced environment and has sedative properties.

DID YOU KNOW?

A common wellness exercise used in paediatrics to help children express their feelings is to ask them to colour in the seven petals of a drawn flower, one for each day of the week. On Monday, the petal colour may be black due to the child not having a good day. Tuesday's petal may be coloured orange because the child feels happy, Wednesday's petal may be coloured blue due to the child feeling calm and relaxed, and so on. This can assist the health professional in determining what happened on Tuesday that did not happen on Monday, etc.

ENVIRONMENTAL COLOURING

One of the more modern aspects of incorporating colour therapy into our everyday lives involves awareness of the physical and psychological effects of colour and how they influence people to behave in certain ways. For example, prisons tend to use soft colours to paint walls, such as pink. This is thought to dampen down incidences of aggression and violence from inmates. Schools often paint walls yellow, orange, or red to stimulate learning. Other colours used in the environment can be seen in Table 8.2.

Table 8.2 Environmental colours.

Colour	Suggested areas best used
Violet	Places of worship Entry areas to clinics and hospitals
Indigo	Bedrooms Treatment rooms
Blue	All rooms except those used for physical activity or play
Green	Depending on the shade, can be used in most areas
Yellow	Activity rooms, i.e. play and study Entrance hallways
Orange	Activity areas Creative areas
Red	Often used in restaurants
Magenta	Lecture spaces Meeting rooms

Clothing

Many colour therapists advocate that the colour of clothing we wear can affect our moods. For example, if you wear a yellow top, you take on the properties of the colour yellow: i.e. happiness and optimism.

DID YOU KNOW?

In the UK, 87% of patients and the public strongly associate the NHS with the colours blue and white (https://www.england.nhs.uk/nhsidentity/identity-guidelines/colours).
In colour therapy, blue is strongly associated with tranquillity and calmness and can be soothing to the eye – perfect for the hospital setting.

Food Colours and Their Benefits

For health, we all need to adhere to a balanced diet that includes food from each of the main groups – carbohydrates; fruit and vegetables; meat, fish, and other proteins; and some fats – in varying proportions. Colour therapists may advocate a

Table 8.3 Food colours and their benefits.

Food colour	Attributes	Associated food
Red	Improves heart and blood health	Strawberries, raspberries, tomatoes
Orange	Promotes collagen growth	Oranges, carrots, mangoes
Yellow	Promotes skin elasticity	Lemon, pineapple, sweetcorn
White	Strengthens the immune system	Cauliflower, garlic, banana
Purple	Powerful antioxidants	Blackberries, blueberries, beetroot
Green	Purifies and detoxifies the body	Cabbage, lettuce, kiwi

rainbow diet for good health. Some colour therapists advocate that this therapy can be used in our eating habits instinctively, such as eating an orange when we have a cold.

A colour therapist may ask a client questions such as 'What is your favourite food? What colours do you have in your fruit bowl and vegetable rack?' Then any lacking colours and/or health problems can be addressed. Table 8.3 shows the food colours and their perceived benefits.

EXERCISE 8.3   Make a Detoxifying Smoothie:

Ingredients:

- ½ cup water
- 1 green apple = contains prebiotics
- ½ cup of frozen pineapple chunks = rich in antioxidants
- ½ frozen banana = good source of potassium
- ½ inch of fresh ginger, peeled and minced = has anti-inflammatory properties
- 1 cup of fresh spinach = contains antioxidants (promotes eye health)
- Small sprig of parsley = rich in antioxidants and has antibacterial properties
- 1 tablespoon fresh lime juice = contains antioxidants and is a great source of vitamin C

Combine all the ingredients in a blender, and blend until smooth. Pour into a glass and drink.

COLOUR THERAPY FOR MOODS AND EMOTIONS

An area of colour therapy looks at how colour can help to induce a particular mood or feeling, evoking certain emotions, and how these neurotransmitters react to release feelings of positivity and happiness. Table 8.4 shows the colours and their associated emotional responses.

What Colour Therapy Can Help with

Evidence suggests that colour therapy can help with many conditions, such as:

- Stress
- Depression
- Aggression
- Hypotension
- Hypertension
- Sleep disorders
- Anxiety

Benefits of Colour Therapy

Some of the benefits of colour therapy are:

Table 8.4 Colours and their emotional response.

Colour	Evokes feelings of:
Red	Increases energy and vitality
Orange	Comforting, warming
Yellow	Mental stimulation
Green	Good for tired nerves and balancing emotions
Blue	Soothing, calming
Purple	Peace, quiet
White	Purifying
Black	Silence, peace
Grey	Inspiring

- **Stress relief** – Certain calming colours, such as blue and green, can have a soothing effect on individuals who are stressed or anxious.
- **Appetite booster** – Warm and stimulating colours may boost the appetite of those struggling with their appetite.
- **Alleviates seasonal affective disorder** – People who suffer from SAD may benefit from warm colours like yellow and orange to alleviate their condition.
- **Energy booster** – Colours such as red and yellow may help to boost energy and make us feel motivated.

HOW EFFECTIVE IS COLOUR THERAPY?

Unfortunately, as with many holistic therapies, some less-than-scrupulous therapists do not use evidence-related practice and may make claims to be able to 'treat' medical conditions. However, some evidence does show that colour therapy can be useful in certain stress and depressive conditions.

EXERCISE 8.4   Colour Breathing

Colour breathing has long been used in the mental health sector. It combines a simple breathing technique (Chapter 4) with visualisation (Chapter 14) and is designed to manage stress and anxiety. This technique involves imagining relaxing colours, such as blue or green, entering the body as you take a deep breath, and then visualising the stress and tension leaving your body as you breathe out, through a colour you don't like as much. This colour breathing technique can be used in both adults and paediatrics:

1   Sit comfortably in a chair with both feet on the ground, or lie on the floor, whichever you prefer. Allow your eyes to close.
2   Take a moment to check out each part of your body, from the top of your head to the tips of your toes. Relax all of your muscles. Notice any tension you are holding, and relax.
3   Bring your awareness to your breathing. Without trying to control your breathing, spend a moment listening to the air flowing in and out. Notice how your breath starts to slow down as you relax.
4   Whilst maintaining your slow, rhythmic, relaxed breath, begin breathing more deeply by ensuring that your abdomen expands as you inhale. Inhale for three seconds through your nose and then exhale for four seconds out of your mouth (if you can manage this). If you feel dizzy, go back to your normal breathing pattern.

5   As you start to feel increasingly relaxed, choose a colour that makes you feel soothed or happy. When you inhale, imagine this colour washing all over you, covering all your stress and tension.

6   Feel that colour travelling through your body parts from the top of your head to the tips of your toes, allowing all the muscles to relax. As you exhale, imagine a colour that you associate with stress or negative feelings leaving your body and, along with it, the anxiety and stress you have built up. Continue to do this for several minutes.

7   When you are ready, slowly start to bring yourself back to the here and now. You might want to wiggle your toes and fingers and then slowly roll your shoulders and neck.

8   When you are ready, open your eyes. Before returning to your day, take a minute or two to appreciate how your body feels.

EXERCISE 8.5   Take a Light Shower

When you feel stressed, a colour therapy stress-relief exercise is to take a **light shower** (and you don't even need to take off any clothes). Stand still for a few moments. Close your eyes, and imagine/visualise a shower of calming green light pouring down all over you. Imagine the soothing green light swirling around you, penetrating your whole body.

When you feel ready, open your eyes and get on with your day.

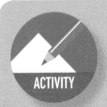

Chapter 8 Activity

Colour Therapy Meditation

Begin by relaxing. Sit down or lie down where you will not be disturbed. Close your eyes and take a few deep breaths.

o   Imagine the stimulating colour of red in your mind. Imagine and enjoy red of all shades – rubies, poppies, apples, red peppers.

o   Red is all around you – immerse yourself in red. Breathe in the colour red, and breathe out the colour red.

o   Breathe in the colour red. and breathe out the colour red.

o   **PAUSE**

o   Now imagine the warming colour of orange in your mind. Imagine and enjoy all the shades of orange – marigolds, carrots, oranges, orange peppers.

o   Orange is all around you – immerse yourself in orange. Breathe in the colour orange, and breathe out the colour orange.

o   Breathe in the colour orange, and breathe out the colour orange.

o   **PAUSE**

o   Now imagine the bright colour of yellow in your mind. Imagine and enjoy all the shades of yellow – lemons, daffodils, yellow peppers, and the leaves turning yellow in autumn.

o   Yellow is all around you – immerse yourself in a sea of yellow. Breathe in the colour yellow, and breathe out the colour yellow.

o   Breathe in the colour yellow, and breathe out the colour yellow.

o   **PAUSE**

o   Now imagine the calming colour of nature – green – in your mind. Imagine and enjoy all the shades of green – plants, leaves, grass, emeralds. Bright greens to pale greens.

o   Green is all around you – immerse yourself in green. Breathe in the colour green, and breathe out the colour green.

o   Breathe in the colour green, and breathe out the colour green.

o   **PAUSE**

o   Now imagine the beautiful colour of blue in your mind. Imagine and enjoy all the shades of blue – water, sky, cornflowers, bluebells.

o   Blue is all around you – immerse yourself in blue. Breathe in the colour blue, and breathe out the colour blue.

o   Breathe in the colour blue, and breathe out the colour blue.

o   **PAUSE**

o   Now imagine the peaceful colour of indigo in your mind. Imagine and enjoy all the shades of indigo – blackberries, blueberries, grapes, plums.

o   Indigo is all around you – immerse yourself in indigo. Breathe in the colour indigo, and breathe out the colour indigo.

o   Breathe in the colour indigo, and breathe out the colour indigo.

o   **PAUSE**

o   Now the colour becomes a lighter shade of indigo: violet.

o   Imagine and enjoy all the shades of violet – violas, amethyst, lavender.

o   Violet is all around you – immerse yourself in violet. Breathe in the colour violet, and breathe out the colour violet.

- o   Breathe in the colour violet, and breathe out the colour violet.
- o   **PAUSE**
- o   Now allow the colour in your imagination to become white.
- o   A pure, breathtaking white.
- o   You are bathed in white.
- o   White consists of all the colours in the spectrum.
- o   **PAUSE**

Slowly return to the here and now. Open your eyes and sit up when ready. In times of stress, try to remember this feeling of calm you are experiencing now.

KEY POINTS

- History of colour therapy
- Colours of the spectrum
- Colour idioms
- How we see colours
- The importance of colours
- Science of colour therapy
- Common colours used during colour therapy
- Environmental colouring
- Colour therapy used in clothing
- Food colours and their benefits
- Colour therapy for moods and emotions
- Tools used in colour therapy sessions
- Benefits of colour therapy
- How effective is colour therapy?

WEB RESOURCES

- **Colour therapy:** https://www.verywellmind.com/color-therapy-definition-types-techniques-and-efficacy-5194910
- **Colour healing:** www.colourtherapyhealing.com
- **Complementary Medical Association:** https://www.the-cma.org.uk/articles/colour-therapy-4209
- **Psychology and colour therapy:** http://www.arttherapyblog.com/online/color-psychology-psychologica-effects-of-colors/#

Chapter 9
· · · · · · · · · · · · · · · · · · ·
AROMATHERAPY

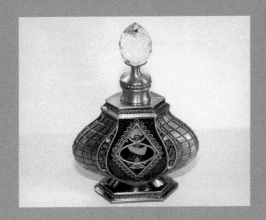

Wellbeing Strategies for Nurses, First Edition. Claire Boyd.
© 2023 John Wiley & Sons Ltd. Published 2023 by John Wiley & Sons Ltd.

LEARNING OUTCOMES

By the end of this chapter, you will have an understanding of how essential oils work, the science of smell, and cautions when using these oils. You will also understand 14 essential oils, how they can be beneficial for stress-related conditions, and how they are used in the hospital setting.

Aromatherapy is a complementary therapy that uses essential oils to improve health and wellbeing. Essential oils are extracted from the stems, leaves, bark, flowers, roots, seeds, resins, or peels of aromatic plants.

DID YOU KNOW?

The use of essential oils dates back over 5000 years to the ancient Greeks and beyond.

HOW DO ESSENTIAL OILS WORK?

The way essential oils work depends on how the oils are used. Many people use essential oils diluted and applied to the skin during a massage; others use them to treat very minor burns, as lavender essential oil can be applied topically to the affected area. Trained aromatherapists may prepare and apply essential oil preparations for certain conditions, as some oils have antibacterial, antifungal, and antimicrobial compounds.

Essential oil molecules are so small that when applied to the skin, they are able to pass through the outer layer of the skin (stratum corneum) and the dermis and into the capillaries and the bloodstream. Absorption also occurs through hair follicles and sweat ducts.

When essential oils are dispersed into the air (diffused), the molecules enter the body through the nose (olfactory system). The next section discusses the science of smell. With every breath, some scent molecules travel to the lungs and are absorbed by the mucous lining of the respiratory pathway. Other molecules reach the alveoli and are transferred into the bloodstream. Using essential oils for wellbeing is called **aromatherapy**, and the impact can be physical as well as emotional.

DID YOU KNOW?

Certain essential oils have been found to affect our brain waves when inhaled, increasing alpha and theta waves. These two types of brain waves promote a sense of relaxation.

THE SCIENCE OF SMELL

Smell begins at the back of the nose, where millions of sensory neurons (called **chemoreceptors**) lie in a strip of tissue called the **olfactory epithelium**. The tips of these cells contain protein receptors that bind odour molecules.

DID YOU KNOW?

Humans have 450 different types of olfactory receptors, perhaps more!

Once an odour molecule binds to a receptor, it initiates an electrical signal that travels from the sensory neurons to the olfactory bulb. The olfactory bulb in the brain sorts sensations into perception. It is part of the limbic system, which includes the amygdala and the hippocampus: structures vital to our behaviour, mood, and memory.

DID YOU KNOW?

Anosmia is the inability to smell. You can be born with anosmia or acquire it due to sinus disease, growths in the nasal passage, viral infections, or head trauma.
As taste and smell are closely related, those with anosmia have impaired taste function.

CAUTIONS AND THERAPEUTIC GUIDELINES

We will only be discussing inhaling essential oils, not applying diluted oils to the skin, as only trained aromatherapists should undertake this task. However, as with any chemical, we need to be aware of a few safety precautions: some oils may be irritating if applied to the skin, and caution should always be taken for anyone pregnant or with certain medical conditions, such as seizures.

ESSENTIAL OILS

There are many essential oils to choose from, but I have chosen 14 oils that we can use for our exercises and in Chapters 17–20. These oils are good for stress-related conditions. Table 9.1 shows the oils with their botanical name, origin, and psychological attributes.

Table 9.1 12 useful essential oils.

Essential oil	Fragrance	Oil from	Psychological attributes
Rosemary Botanical name: *Rosmarinus officinalis*	Fresh, penetrating, herby, with warm woody notes	Leaves and twigs	Helps with concentration and stress-related disorders
Sweet orange Botanical name: *Citrus sinensis*	Sweet, fresh, fruity, tangy	Peel	Stress-relieving, nervous tension

Table 9.1 (*Continued*)

Essential oil	Fragrance	Oil from	Psychological attributes
Ylang-ylang Botanical name: *Cananga odorata*	Exotic, Oriental, heady, musky, slightly spicy, floral	Flowers	Deeply relaxing, destressing, soothes troubled mind and spirit
Lemon Botanical name: *Citrus limonum*	Bright, fresh, sweet	Fruit peel	Antidepressant, uplifting, improves the feeling of wellbeing
Geranium Botanical name: *Pelargonium graveolens*	Very sweet, rose-like, slightly minty, lemony	Leaves	Good for nervous tension and stress-related conditions
Pine Botanical name: *Pinus sylvestris*	Fresh, woody, penetrating, camphoraceous	Pine needles	Fatigue, nervous exhaustion, stress-related conditions
Lime Botanical name: *Citrus aurantifolia*	Fresh, bitter, citrus, green, fruity, clean	Peel of unripe fruit or crushed whole, ripe fruit	Uplifting, nervous exhaustion
Lavender Botanical name: *Lavandula angustifolia*	Floral with woody undertones	Flower tops	Depression, headache, insomnia, nervous tension, stress
Peppermint Botanical name: *Mentha piperita*	Fresh, sharp and penetrating, minty, cooling	Leaves	Mental fatigue, nervous stress, headache
Tea tree Botanical name: *Melaleuca alternifolia*	Strongly medicinal, pungent, clean, green, fresh	Leaves and twigs	Vitalising, fresh, lifts the spirit
Eucalyptus Botanical name: *Eucalyptus globulus*	Strong, fresh, medicinal, sharp, with a woody undertone	Leaves and young twigs	Clearing, fresh and bright, gives a feeling of space
Bergamot Botanical name: *Citrus bergamia*	Fresh, soft, citrus, sweet, slightly spicy-floral, green	Peel of the fruit	Anxiety, depression, stress-related conditions; uplifting qualities

Table 9.2 shows two other very expensive essential oils that I like to use. My family usually buy these for me for Christmas or birthdays.

Table 9.3 shows the properties of these oils. The meanings of the terms can be viewed in Appendix C.

Table 9.2 Two expensive essential oils.

Rose Botanical name: *Rosa centifolia*	Honey-sweet, very floral, musky, spicy	Petals	Helps with feelings of depression, insomnia, headaches, and stress-related complaints
Sandalwood Botanical name: *Santalum album*	Soft, amber, sweet, rich with warm, woody, spicy undertones	Wood	Deeply relaxing and calming; good for anxiety, depression, and insomnia

Table 9.3 Properties of essential oils.

Rosemary	Analgesic, antimicrobial, astringent, carminative, choleretic, cicatrizant, cordial, diaphoretic, digestive, diuretic, emmenagogue, fungicidal, hepatic, hypertensor, restorative, rubefacient, stimulant, stomachic, sudorific, tonic
Sweet orange	Antidepressant, anti-inflammatory, antiseptic, bactericidal, carminative, choleretic, digestive, fungicidal, hypotensor, sedative (to the nervous system), stimulant
Ylang-ylang	Aphrodisiac, antidepressant, anti-infectious, antiseborrheic, antiseptic, euphoric, hypotensive, nervine, regulator, sedative (nervous system), stimulant (circulatory system), tonic
Lemon	Anti-anaemic, antimicrobial, antirheumatic, anticlerotic, antiseptic, antispasmodic, antitoxic, astringent, bactericide, carminative, cicatrizant, depurative, diaphoretic, diuretic, febrifuge, hemostatic, hypotensive, insecticide, rubefacient, tonic, vermifuge
Geranium	Antihemorrhagic, anti-inflammatory, antiseptic, astringent, cicatrizant, deodorant, diuretic, fungicidal, hemostatic, stimulant (adrenal cortex and lymphatic system), styptic, tonic, vermifuge, vulnerary
Pine	Antimicrobial, antineuralgic, antirheumatic, antiscorbutic, antiseptic, antiviral, bactericidal, balsamic, cholagogue, choleretic, deodorant, diuretic, expectorant, hypertensor, insecticide, restorative, rubefacient, stimulant (circulatory and nervous system), vermifuge

Table 9.3 (*Continued*)

Lime	Antirheumatic, antiscorbutic, antiseptic, antiviral, aperitif, bactericidal, febrifuge, restorative, tonic
Lavender	Analgesic, anticonvulsive, antimicrobial, antirheumatic, antiseptic, antispasmodic Antitoxic, carminative, cholagogue, choleretic, cytophylactic, deodorant, diuretic, emmenagogue, hypotensor, insecticide, nervine, parasiticide, rubefacient, sedative, stimulant, sudorific, tonic, vermifuge, vulnerary
Peppermint	Analgesic, anti-inflammatory, antimicrobial, antiphlogistic, antipruritic, antiseptic, antispasmodic, antiviral, astringent, diaphoretic, carminative, cephalic, cordial, emmenagogue, expectorant, febrifuge, hepatic, nervine, stomachic, sudorific, vasoconstrictor, vermifuge
Tea tree	Anti-infectious, anti-inflammatory, antiseptic, antiviral, bactericidal, balsamic, cicatrizant, diaphoretic, expectorant, fungicidal, immunostimulant, parasiticide, vulnerary
Eucalyptus	Analgesic, antineuralgic, antiseptic, antiviral, cicatrizant, decongestant, deodorant, depurative, diuretic, expectorant, febrifuge, hypoglycaemic, parasiticide, rubefacient, stimulant, vermifuge, vulnerary, insecticide
Bergamot	Analgesic, anthelmintic, antiseptic, antispasmodic, antitoxic, carminative, digestive, diuretic, deodorant, febrifuge, parasiticide, rubefacient, stimulant, stomachic, tonic, vermifuge, vulnerary, insecticide
Rose	Antidepressant, antiphlogistic, antiseptic, antispasmodic, antiviral, bactericidal, choleretic, cicatrizant, depurative, hemostatic, hepatic, appetite regulator, sedative, stomachic, tonic
Sandalwood	Antidepressant, antiphlogistic, antiseptic, antispasmodic, aphrodisiac, astringent, bactericidal, carminative, cicatrizant, diuretic, expectorant, fungicidal, insecticide, sedative, tonic

DID YOU KNOW?

It can take 10–20 pounds of lavender flowers to produce 1 ounce of lavender essential oil and 2000 rose petals to yield just one drop of rose essential oil.

EXERCISE 9.1   Scenting Pine Cones

Go for a walk, and pick up some pine cones. Clean them with warm water. Then soak the cones in a little water (enough to completely cover them) in a bowl with 30–40 drops of pine essential oil (or any other smell you like – orange, geranium, and sandalwood are good). After a day or two, shake them off and place them around your home. When they are fully dry, I like to put them by my computer so that the warmth gently releases the smells.

Any leftover water can be used in a vaporiser.

Using Essential Oils in Vaporisers

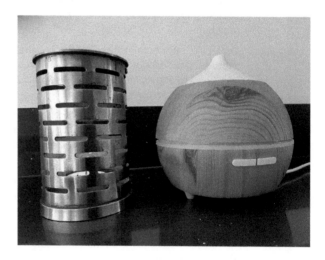

Essential oils can be added to tea-light diffusers, electric diffusers, and vaporisers. The essential oils of your choice are added to water in or on the diffuser, and as the water warms, the scent is released. Diffusers have the added benefit of the healing properties being released into the environment. During the first episode of the coronavirus pandemic, we used a lot of antiviral essential oils around the home.

If you don't have a diffuser, vaporiser, or tea-light holder, you can make your own reed diffuser.

EXERCISE 9.2   How to Make a Reed Diffuser

1   Find a small narrow-necked glass or ceramic bottle or jar (you can recycle something).
2   Fill ¼ of the bottle with either grapeseed oil or water with 5 ml vodka.
3   Add approximately 40 drops of your chosen essential oils (or blend).
4   Place 6–8 reeds in the liquid and allow to saturate; then take them out and place the opposite ends into the bottle. The reeds should stick well above the bottle/vase you are using.
5   Rotate the reeds once a week, and add 5–10 drops more of your chosen essential oils when the mixture loses its smell.

Note: You can buy reed diffusers very cheaply online or use bamboo cooking skewers with the pointed ends cut off. I tend to recycle reeds from diffusers brought for me as Christmas presents, etc.

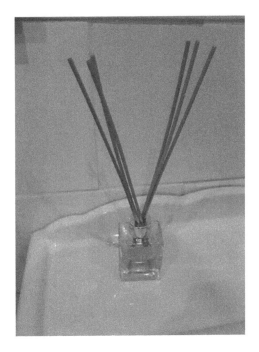

Blends for Reed Diffusers

You can add a mix of your favourite oils to your reed diffuser. Some of my favourites are shown in Table 9.4.

Table 9.4 Essential oil blends to use in a reed diffuser.

Sweet dreams blend	60 drops lavender in grapeseed oil or water/vodka
Citrus grove blend	30 drops lemon 30 drops sweet orange in grapeseed oil or water/vodka
A walk in Tuscany blend	30 drops lemon 30 drops rosemary in grapeseed oil or water/vodka
Good morning blend	30 drops peppermint 30 drops rosemary in grapeseed oil or water/vodka
Clean air blend	20 drops sweet orange 20 drops lime 20 drops peppermint in grapeseed oil or water/vodka
Herbal bouquet	40 drops lavender 20 drops rosemary in grapeseed oil or water/vodka

EXERCISE 9.3   Enhance Sleep

If you want to sleep like a baby, put a few drops of lavender essential oil on your pillow to help stimulate positive signals in the brain, calming the mind and enhancing sleep.

This is why so many commercial sleep remedies contain lavender oil.

USING ESSENTIAL OILS IN THE HEALTHCARE SETTING

Essential oils are used increasingly in the healthcare setting to help with pain, anxiety, and nausea, amongst other things:

Pain: Studies show that aromatherapy seems to have beneficial effects on pain severity and positively influences mood and quality of life. It is mainly used to assist with postoperative pain and obstetric and gynecologic pain. In studies, lavender essential oil has been shown to have both analgesic and anti-inflammatory effects.

Anxiety: Studies have looked at the use of essential oils to decrease anxiety in the postoperative period. Other randomised trials have shown that certain essential oils, used alone or concomitantly with mindfulness meditation, reduce general anxiety levels: e.g. Lavandula, Rosa damascene, *Citrus aurantium*, peppermint, and chamomilla. Other studies revealed that the use of lavender oil on patients undergoing haemodialysis decreased fatigue and anxiety levels.

Nausea: Studies have found that essential oils can be used to manage postoperative nausea and vomiting, as well as other gastrointestinal issues, such as dyspepsia and irritable bowel syndrome. Other randomised trials with essential oils with patients who reported nausea in the post-anaesthesia period found significant changes in nausea levels and requests for anti-emetic medications in patients using ginger essential oil or lavender oils.

EXERCISE 9.4 Sweet-Smelling Underwear

Put a few drops of your chosen essential oil onto a cotton wool ball, and place this in your underwear or sock drawer. Every time you open the drawer, you will get a pleasant whiff of the scent.

ESSENTIAL OILS AND STRESS RELIEF

Studies on essential oils have suggested that the best oils to use for certain circumstances are as shown in Table 9.5.

Table 9.5 Essential oils used for certain conditions.

Relaxation	Lavender	When a 3% dilution of lavender essential oil was sprayed on clothing, a study in 2013 suggested it reduced workplace stress.
Sleep	Chamomile	A study in 2018 found that chamomile helped reduce anxiety symptoms and increased morning cortisol levels.
Meditation	Orange	A 2012 study found that participants who inhaled sweet orange essential oil did not have an increase in anxiety or tension during an anxiety-inducing situation, unlike those who inhaled a control aroma (tea tree oil) or a placebo.
Anxiety	Sandalwood	A study in 2006 found that sandalwood oil was effective at reducing anxiety amongst participants.
Stress	Clary sage	A study in 2014 found that clary sage was effective at decreasing cortisol levels and produced an antidepressant-like effect for menopausal women when inhaled.

(*Continued*)

Table 9.5 (*Continued*)

Mood lifter	Lemon	According to a 2005 study, lemon oil significantly enhanced the attention level, concentration, cognitive performance, and mood of students during the learning process.
Diffusing	Bergamot	A 2017 study found that inhaling bergamot essential oil for 15 minutes improved positive feelings of participants in the waiting room of a mental health treatment centre.
Depression	Jasmine	A 2013 study examined the effects on brain activity when participants inhaled jasmine oil. The researchers concluded that the stimulating and activating effect of jasmine oil could be useful for relieving depression and improving mood.
Rest	Ylang-ylang	Preliminary research from 2006 suggested that ylang-ylang can help decrease blood pressure and create a relaxing effect.

EXERCISE 9.5   Quick-Fix Stress Relief

When you are feeling stressed, put a few drops of lavender essential oil onto a clean tissue for inhalation throughout the day.

Chapter 9 Activity

ACTIVITY

Make Your Own Spray Air Freshener Using Essential Oils

You will need:

- A small spray/mist bottle (try to recycle a previously used perfume bottle)
- 2 tablespoons vodka (or 3 tablespoons witch hazel)
- 6 tablespoons filtered water
- 25 drops of your chosen essential oils

1 Put the alcohol/witch hazel and water into the spray bottle.
2 Add the essential oils.
3 Let the mixture sit for five minutes, and then shake well.
4 Spritz around your room.
5 Shake the bottle each time before use.

Suggested oils to use: orange, lavender, or peppermint; or make up a combination of your own – orange and peppermint work well together.

KEY POINTS

- What is aromatherapy?
- How do essential oils work?
- The science of smell
- Cautions and therapeutic guidelines for using essential oils
- The chemistry of essential oils
- Essential oils – botanical names, origins and psychological attributes
- Using essential oils in vaporisers
- How to make a reed diffuser
- Using essential oils in the healthcare setting
- Essential oils for stress relief
- Essential oil room air fresheners

WEB RESOURCES

Sleep: https://essentialoilexperts.com/essential-oils-for-sleep
Aromatherapy used in hospitals: https://www.isbewonders.com/aromatherapy-in-hospitals-and-suggested-uses

Chapter 10

SHARING
WITH FRIENDS

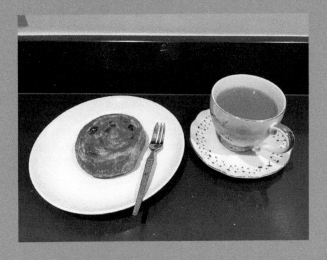

Wellbeing Strategies for Nurses, First Edition. Claire Boyd.
© 2023 John Wiley & Sons Ltd. Published 2023 by John Wiley & Sons Ltd.

LEARNING OUTCOMES

By the end of this chapter, you will have an understanding of how friendships can enrich our lives and reduce our stress and how to nurture these friendships. You will also be aware of the Scandinavian life philosophies for happiness and the benefits of therapeutic baking.

Friendships can have a major impact on our health and wellbeing, with the right friends being good for our health. Social contact is one of the most important ways of relieving stress. As we all live busy lives, it can be all too easy to let our friendships slide, but studies are now showing how important it is to have friendships to improve our mental health.

FRIENDS ENRICH OUR LIVES

Whether we have an intimate circle of friends or would like to enlarge that circle of social support, surrounding ourselves we people we can trust, who are supportive and empathic listeners, helps us to cope with life's trials and reduce our stress.

Studies have also shown that older adults who have meaningful relationships and good social support networks are likely to live longer than their peers with fewer connections.

DID YOU KNOW?

A study by the *American Journal of Epidemiology* (2017) found that people who use Facebook showed signs of lower wellbeing. Social media can detract from face-to-face relationships and more meaningful in-person activities. It can also increase sedentary behaviour and hurt your self-esteem because it causes you to compare yourself to others in a negative way (https://academic.oup.com/aje/article/185/3/203/2915143).

As we can see, social media 'friendships' don't count, but healthy friendships can help to reduce our stress, as described in Table 10.1.

Table 10.1 Ways in which friends can help to reduce our stress.

Friends reduce stress.	Research has shown that during stressful times, being around a friend decreases our levels of the stress hormone cortisol.
Friends make us healthier.	Friends can make us healthier by encouraging us to avoid or change unhealthy lifestyle habits.
Friends can help our mental agility.	Research has shown that a 10-minute chat on a social topic can boost executive function, the type of mental agility that helps us to solve problems.
Friends can make us laugh.	Laughter is good for us (see Chapter 11); it improves mood, reduces stress, and may even boost our immune system. Friends have the ability to make us laugh.
Friends can help us to live longer.	Research has found that people with strong social ties live longer than those without.
Friends can help us not to feel lonely.	Without friends, loneliness and social isolation can affect our mental and physical wellbeing. Friends can help avoid this isolation.
Friends can provide emotional support.	Emotional support is an important benefit of relationships. Our friends might support us by listening, validating our feelings, doing nice things for us, and helping distract us when we are sad or upset.
Friends can help with our personal development.	Friends can help us when we want to make positive life changes and cheer us on and support us. This encouragement can boost our self-confidence, increasing our chances of success with our goals
Friends can give us a sense of belonging.	Developing and maintaining close friendships can help foster a feeling of security and belonging. Even when our friends are scattered over several cities (or countries), we still know we have these connections and trusted friends who have our backs.
Friends can help support us through challenging times.	We all have challenges throughout life. Studies have shown that friendship increases our ability to recover from distressing life events, such as divorce, death, pandemics, and unemployment.

HOW TO NURTURE FRIENDSHIPS

Developing and maintaining healthy friendships involves give and take. Sometimes you are the one giving support, and at other times, you may be on the receiving end. To nurture your friendships, consider some of the tips in Table 10.2.

Table 10.2 Tips to nurture your friendships.

Be kind.	This most basic behaviour remains the core of successful relationships.
Be a good listener.	When friends share details of hard times or difficult experiences, really listen to what they are saying and be empathetic.
Open up.	Build intimacy with your friends by opening up about yourself, as this helps deepen your connection.
Show that you can be trusted.	Being responsible, reliable, and dependable is key to forming strong friendships.
Make yourself available.	Make an effort to see your friends regularly, and contact them between catch-ups.
Go to social events if you can (even if you don't always feel like it).	You may feel tempted to stay at home, but sometimes you need to make an effort to go out with friends.

EXERCISE 10.1   Random Acts of Kindness

Show a friend a random act of kindness. Choose one of these suggestions, and implement it today. Some of these can be acts of kindness to your friends or complete strangers (but obviously not telling a stranger how much you love them)!

- **Give a compliment.** It can be a big or a small compliment. This can make someone feel confident.
- **Sort out some belongings you no longer use, and give them to charity.** This can be very cathartic and appreciated by the charity.
- **Give someone a call who you haven't spoken to for a while.** This will make them feel special, knowing that you are thinking about them.
- **Give your time.** Show others that you are there for them. Your time is the most valuable thing you can give someone.

- **If you have a special someone, tell them how much you love them**. Let them know how happy you are to have them in your life.
- **Say thank you to someone**. In our haste, we often forget to do this. By saying thank you, we can make others feel appreciated.
- **Give a gift**. It does not have to be a large gift (perhaps some baking). It just lets them know you are thinking about them, which will make them feel good.
- **Just be nice**. Always be aware of your words and actions.

STRIVE TOWARDS HAPPINESS

We all want to be happy in life. For inspiration, we can look to the Scandinavian approach to life; according to the World Happiness Report, Scandinavian countries, despite their long, hard, cold winters, have been rated as the happiest countries in the world for several years running. The reason has been cited as Scandinavian life philosophies. So, what are these life philosophies? And can you use any of these philosophies in your life? Table 10.3 shows the five most popular Scandinavian life philosophies that can make you happier.

We can all incorporate fika into our lives. Combined with the therapeutic benefits of baking, it is a marriage made in heaven.

Table 10.3 Five Scandinavian life philosophies that can make you happier.

Fika (Sweden)	**Fika literally translates to 'coffee break', but it incorporates the philosophy of finding inner peace and altering attitudes to life in general. Whereas we might take coffee for the caffeine burst to wake ourselves up, the fika concept is about coffee being drunk to help us slow us down, breathe out, and relax for a moment. Drinking tea and coffee is mostly to savour the moment, enjoy your life, and dissociate from your daily stress. Fika is about giving you peace and allowing you to retreat from pressure.**
Friluftsliv (Norway)	**Friluftsliv is a concept that focuses on fostering not only your spiritual wellbeing but also your physical health. It translates as 'free air life' and is about spending more time outside and feeling more connected to nature. The concept is that a healthy person is a much happier person.**

(Continued)

Table 10.3 (*Continued*)

Hygge (Denmark)	Hygge refers to the practice of appreciating life, no matter what, and being positive in everything you do and say. It can be translated to 'cosiness of the soul' and is like the feeling of being tucked up in a blanket next to a roaring fire with a loved one, with a hot drink. Hygge is about allowing yourself to indulge in things that make you feel good and that you enjoy for your wellbeing.
Lagom (Sweden)	Lagom can be translated as 'optimal' or 'moderate'. This concept is about everything in moderation and not being extreme in your beliefs or your actions – being flexible and tolerant when it comes to hearing other people. Lagom is about finding the right balance that can lead to maximum enjoyment.
Lykke Danmark and (Norway)	Lykke is the Danish and Norwegian word for 'happiness'. Happiness may take the form of togetherness, money, health, freedom, trust, and kindness. Lykke is about finding your joy.

THERAPEUTIC BAKING

Baking is not just about enjoying yummy treats: studies have shown that baking also has therapeutic value, which helps to ease depression and anxiety. Table 10.4 shows five reasons baking has been cited as being good for mental health.

Table 10.4 Five reasons baking is good for mental health.

Cooking is meditative.	Baking is an activity that takes up your whole attention and can have a calming, meditative quality. The process of weighing out the ingredients creates a space in the mind and eases out negative thinking processes.
Baking stimulates the senses.	The feel of rubbing flour and butter, the sound of the whisk, and the smell of the finished product – all these experiences stimulate the senses, which in turn increases feel-good endorphins.

Table 10.4 (*Continued*)

Nourishing activities feel good.	Any sort of food preparation, including baking, is ultimately about nourishing ourselves and others. This brings in the feel-good factor.
Baking is creative.	Studies have found a strong connection between creative expression and overall wellbeing. Bake what you want, and decorate it how you want – express yourself!
Baking makes other people happy.	You can give away or share your creations to make others happy – which in turn will make you happy.

So, turn on the oven, get out the weighing scales, and start baking. The next three exercises are some recipes to get you started. (Note that you may wish to look up some less-calorific delights.)

EXERCISE 10.2   Chocolate Chip Cookies

Ingredients:	Method:
460 grams melted butter 440 grams brown sugar 400 grams granulated sugar 4 large eggs 1 tablespoon vanilla extract 625 grams plain flour 2 teaspoons baking powder 700 grams chocolate chips	1 Heat oven to 190 °C (170 °C fan). 2 In a large bowl, whisk together the brown sugar, granulated sugar, and melted butter until evenly combined. 3 Add the whisked eggs and vanilla extract, mixing until smooth. 4 Add flour and baking powder, folding the mixture until it forms a soft dough. 5 Fold in the chocolate chips until evenly combined.

6	Using an ice cream scoop, scoop six balls of the dough onto a baking tray lined with baking parchment.
7	Bake for 12 minutes.

This recipe makes approximately 30 chewy cookies.

EXERCISE 10.3   Classic Scones

Ingredients:	Method	
225 grams self-rising flour (and a little extra for rolling) 50 grams cold butter, cubed 150 mL whole milk	1	Preheat oven to 220 °C (fan 200 °C), Gas 7.
	2	Sift the flour (and a pinch of salt) into a large bowl.
	3	Using your fingertips, rub in the butter until it looks like bread crumbs.
	4	Make a well in the centre of the crumb mix, and pour in the milk. Using a knife, quickly bring the mixture together to form a soft dough.
	5	Knead briefly on a lightly floured surface until smooth, and then roll out to a thickness of about 2 cm.
	6	Using a 5 cm plain metal cutter, stamp out rounds (do not twist).
	7	Knead up any leftover dough, and reuse to make more scones.
	8	Place the scones on a baking tray lined with baking parchment.
	9	Bake for 15 minutes until well-risen and golden.
	10	Transfer to a wire rack, and leave to cool.

Serve with thick cream and jam.

EXERCISE 10.4   Flapjacks

Ingredients:	Method
125 grams butter (and a little extra for greasing the baking tin) 90 grams golden syrup 90 grams light muscovado sugar 250 grams rolled oats 	1 Preheat oven to 180°C (fan 160°C), Gas 4. 2 Lightly butter a baking tin (approx. 20×30 cm), and line it with baking parchment. 3 Combine the butter, syrup, and sugar in a large saucepan, and heat gently until the ingredients have melted and dissolved. 4 Stir in the oats, and mix well. 5 Pour into the prepared tin, and smooth the surface. 6 Bake for about 30 minutes. 7 Leave to cool in the tin for about five minutes, and then mark into 24 fingers. 8 Leave to cool completely, and then cut out and remove from tin. You can add dried fruit or nuts for a variation.

DID YOU KNOW?

It has been said that there are fewer better ways to let off steam than kneading dough – you can really unleash your frustrations and ease your stress for the moment!

Chapter 10 Activity

ACTIVITY

We have seen the benefits of how friends can help us to reduce our stress. We have also seen how baking can be therapeutic. So, call a few friends and invite them round for a catch-up. Bake a few cookies, scones, and flapjacks, and put the kettle on (or rustle up some cocktails) – but remember the concept of lagom (moderation)!

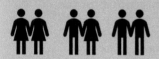

KEY POINTS

- Friends enrich our lives.
- Friends help to reduce our stress.
- How to nurture friendships
- Happiness
- Scandinavian life philosophies that can make us happier
- The benefits of therapeutic baking

WEB RESOURCES

- **Baking and mental health:** https://www.goodnet.org/articles/5-reasons-baking-good-for-mental-health
- **Friendship and stress reduction**: https://www.ornish.com/zine/why-spending-time-with-friends-will-lower-your-

stress, https://www.thepip.com/en-gb/2016/07/
five-ways-your-friends-can-help-you-reduce-stress,
https://www.huffingtonpost.co.uk/entry/best-friend-
stress-levels_n_981080, https://academic.oup.com/aje/
article/185/3/203/2915143

- **Scandinavian life philosophies:** http://www.cavatinala.
  com/5-scandinavian-life-philosophies-that-can-make-
  you-happier

Chapter 11

· · · · · · · · · · · · · · · · · · · ·

HUMOUR THERAPY

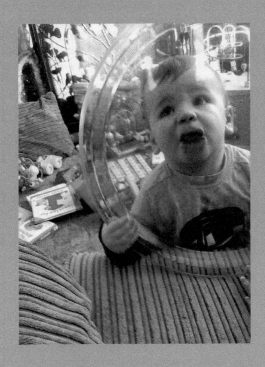

Wellbeing Strategies for Nurses, First Edition. Claire Boyd.
© 2023 John Wiley & Sons Ltd. Published 2023 by John Wiley & Sons Ltd.

LEARNING OUTCOMES

By the end of this chapter, you will have an understanding of the physical, mental, and social benefits of laughter and laughter therapies used for stress relief. You will also be aware of using humour, how to bring more laughter into your life, and how to develop your sense of humour. In addition, you will be able to practice a variety of laughter therapy exercises.

Children can find the humour in many situations – a burb or passing wind can cause a full-blown set of the giggles! As we get older, life often encroaches on us: money worries, job worries, and relationship concerns, to name just a few issues. The burdens we carry can bring us down. We may find life joyless and bleak. Laughter therapy is a recognised 'treatment' for those suffering from depression. I always incorporate humour in my teaching for healthcare professionals to add a little fun to the often intense lectures.

DID YOU KNOW?

My therapist told me the way to achieve true inner peace is to finish what I start.
So far, I've finished two bags of Maltesers and a chocolate fudge cake – I feel better already. Burp!

THE BENEFITS OF LAUGHTER

Laughter is actually good for your health. According to studies, laughter activates the ventromedial prefrontal cortex, releasing endorphins, which as we know are the chemicals responsible for feelings of pleasure and satisfaction and for blocking pain. In the medical profession, laughter as a therapy has become popular in helping people cope with stress, anxiety, and depression. Table 11.1 shows some of the benefits of laughter for your health.

Table 11.1 The benefits of laughter.

Laughter relaxes the whole body.	A really good, hearty laugh relieves physical tension and stress and leaves your muscles relaxed for up to 45 minutes afterwards.
Laughter boosts the immune system.	Laughter improves your resistance to disease by decreasing stress hormones and increasing immune cells and infection-fighting antibodies.
Laughter triggers the release of endorphins.	Endorphins are the body's natural feel-good chemicals. They promote the overall sense of wellbeing and can even temporarily relieve pain.
Laughter protects the heart.	Laughter can protect you against heart attacks and other cardiovascular problems by improving the function of blood vessels and increasing blood flow.
Laughter burns calories.	A study found that laughing for 10–15 minutes a day can burn off approximately 40 calories. Over a year, this could equate to 3 or 4 pounds in weight.
Laughter helps to diffuse difficult situations.	Looking at the funny side can put problems into perspective and may even diffuse conflict faster. Beware, as this could also go the other way and make the situation worse!
Laughter may help you live longer.	A study of patients, including some with cancer, found that those with a strong sense of humour outlived those who didn't laugh so much.

The physical, mental, and social benefits of laughter and humour can be seen in Table 11.2.

Table 11.2 The physical, mental, and social benefits of humour.

Physical health benefits	• Boosts immunity • Lowers stress hormones • Decreases pain • Relaxes your muscles • Prevents heart disease
Mental health benefits	• Adds joy to life • Eases anxiety and tension • Relieves stress • Improves mood • Strengthens resilience
Social benefits	• Strengthens relationships • Enhances teamwork • Helps diffuse conflict (in some situations) • Promotes group bonding

DID YOU KNOW?

Doctor (Hunter) Patch Adams was a medical doctor (and clown and activist) who believed that laughter, joy, and creativity are integral to the healing process.
Note that this is not a picture of Doctor Patch Adams!

LAUGHTER THERAPIES FOR STRESS RELIEF

There are numerous therapies related to laughter and stress, and they have led to the creation of new therapies used by mental health professionals, doctors, psychiatrists, and others to help patients experiencing emotional, physical, and mental health conditions:

Humour therapy – Humour therapy uses books, television, movies, stories, etc., to encourage patients to share entertaining stories about their lives.

Clown therapy – Many children's hospitals use clowns who perform by singing, juggling, performing magic tricks, etc. The positive effects include reducing feelings of pain and heightening stimulation of children's immune systems. A word of caution: some individuals suffer from coulrophobia.

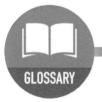

GLOSSARY

Coulrophobia
A fear (phobia) of clowns.

Meditation with laughter – This meditation is similar to mindfulness (see Chapter 13), with laughter inducing the person to enjoy the present moment. This laughter therapy may begin with stretching, then laughing, and then a period of silent meditation with deep breathing and focusing on the moment.

Laughter yoga and laughter clubs – This laughter therapy usually includes breathing exercises, yoga, and stretching – all accompanied by laughter.

DID YOU KNOW?

Scientists have estimated that 100 laughs are equivalent to a 10-minute session on a rowing machine.
   I know which exercise I would prefer!

HUMOUR AND A WORD OF CAUTION

We don't all find the same things funny, as humour is subjective. During lectures in my training sessions, I would sometimes throw in what I thought was a funny remark – but you could see the tumbleweed rolling across the lecture theatre! So, you need to be careful that you don't offend anyone and also remember that what you think is funny, others may not. An example is the top 25 comedy movies of all time, according to Blu-Ray.com, most of which I would give a miss (see Table 11.3). The movies I think are funniest are *Father of the Bride, Mars Attack, Paul, The Birdcage, Little Miss Sunshine*; and I watch *Elf* with my grandsons.

Table 11.3 The top 25 comedy movies of all time.

1	*Dumb and Dumber*
2	*Monty Python and the Holy Grail*
3	*Office Space*
4	*Ghostbusters*

(*Continued*)

Table 11.3 (*Continued*)

5	*Anchorman: The Legend of Ron Burgundy*
6	*The Hangover*
7	*The Jerk*
8	*Ferris Bueller's Day Off*
9	*Caddyshack*
10	*National Lampoon's Animal House*
11	*Blazing Saddles*
12	*The Big Lebowski*
13	*Spaceballs*
14	*Hot Fuzz*
15	*Planes, Trains, and Automobiles*
16	*Ace Ventura: Pet Detective*
17	*Shaun of the Dead*
18	*Airplane*
19	*The 40-Year-Old Virgin*
20	*Step Brothers*
21	*Knocked Up*
22	*National Lampoon's Christmas Vacation*
23	*Groundhog Day*
24	*Dr. Strangelove or: How I Learned to Stop Worrying and Love the Bomb*
25	*Young Frankenstein*

EXERCISE 11.1 Watch A Comedy

On your next day off, snuggle up on the couch, and put on a comedy movie. You can do this on your own or with a couple of friends. Wrap yourself in a blanket if you want, and gather a few snacks and drinks.

DID YOU KNOW?

It's possible to laugh even if you can't find anything funny: **simulated** laughter can be just as beneficial as the real thing. Also, hearing others laugh can often trigger genuine laughter. I'm giving you this information before you do the next exercise and groan!

EXERCISE 11.2 Read Some Jokes

Spend a few moments reading these jokes.

What did the mayonnaise say when the refrigerator door was opened?	Close the door. I'm dressing
Receptionist: Doctor, the Invisible Man has come to see you. He does not have an appointment.	Doctor: Tell him I can't see him.
Exaggerations have become an epidemic.	They went up by a million percent last year!
What do you call a bear with no ears?	B!
What do you call a sad coffee?	Despresso
What sound does a nut make when it sneezes?	Ca-shew!
I was wondering why the ball was getting bigger.	Then it hit me!
Philip, do you think I am a bad parent?	My name is Simon!
What do you call a Frenchman wearing sandals?	Phillipe Phillope
The past, present, and future walked into a bar.	It was tense.
Have you heard about the new restaurant called Karma?	There is no menu; you just get what you deserve!
Do you have a date for Valentine's Day?	Yes – it's February 14th!

Never laugh at your partner's choices.

I have a very secure job.

You are one of them!

There's nobody else who would want it!

What is an ironing board?

A surf board that gave up on its dream and went to work.

Doctor: Your partner is in hospital.

Me: How is she?

Doctor: She is critical.

Me: Oh, you get used to that!

Teacher: Why didn't you do your homework?

Pupil: My dad is in hospital

(One day later)
Teacher: Why have you still not done your homework?

Pupil: My dad is still in hospital.

Pupil: Yes

Gosh! It must be serious!

Pupil: He's the doctor!

(One week later.)
Teacher: Let me guess! Your father is still in hospital. How come?

I called my parents and told them not to worry, but I'm in hospital.

My mother said, 'This wasn't funny the first time you said it – you're the flaming doctor!'

Covid medical 'experts' are such liars! They said after you've had your injections, masks were all you needed to go shopping.

But when I got to the store, everyone was wearing clothes!

I took a urine test at the hospital yesterday.

Boy, my kleptomania is out of control!

TWITTER JOKES

These next jokes are the top 10 jokes, according to people on Twitter. As I've said before, humour is very subjective – but you may find them funny!

1. As we approached the airport, the pilot started banking. A ridiculous time for a career change, I felt!

2   My wife is threatening to leave me because of my constant celebrity name-dropping. David Beckham warned me that this might happen.

3   I asked my dad once, 'Where were you when you heard that Kennedy had been shot?'. He said, 'HE'S BEEN SHOT?!'

4   65% of mathematicians have a sense of humour. The other 45% don't find jokes like this funny.

5   Whoever came up with naming birds really missed a trick by not calling a baby pigeon a smidgen.

6   The first rule of Pirate Club: Pirate Club is for private ears only.

7   If Elvis was alive today, he'd probably be dead now.

8   Me, singing: 'Go to sleep, go to sleep little baby'. Policewoman: 'I said do you have an alibi!'

9   (As olive oil prices rise in the drought): Now I'm losing the huile d'olive.

10   I wouldn't say Jet Set Willie was completely ZX, but he was certainly on the ZX Spectrum.

HOW TO BRING MORE LAUGHTER INTO YOUR LIFE

Babies begin to smile during their first weeks of life and can laugh aloud within months. As adults, we may have lost the ability to laugh as much as we should. We can kick-start the process by:

Smile. Smiling is the beginning of laughter and is contagious. Make an effort to smile, and notice the effect on others.

Count your blessings. Sit down and make a list. This will help to distance yourself from negative thoughts that block humour and laughter.

When you hear laughter, move towards it. More often, people are very happy to share something funny because it gives them an opportunity to laugh again and feed off the humour you find in it.

Spend time with fun and playful people. Seek out people who like to laugh and make others laugh. These are usually the type of people who often find humour in everyday situations.

Bring humour into the conversation. Ask people, 'What's the funniest thing that happened to you today? This week? This year?'

Exercise 11.3   Visit A Comedy Club

When you next get paid, and if you can afford it, invite friends and co-workers out to a comedy club.

DID YOU KNOW?

Did you hear about the scarecrow who won an award?
He was out standing in his field!
(Thanks for the joke, Owen – told you I'd put it in the book!)

HOW TO DEVELOP YOUR SENSE OF HUMOUR

It may not be about developing your sense of humour; you may just have to remember how to laugh. When we are tired, stressed, and unhappy with life, sometimes we need a little reminder to find the joy:

- **Laugh at yourself.** The best way to take yourself less seriously is to share your embarrassing moments with others.
- **Attempt to laugh at situations rather than moan about them**. Look for humour even in difficult situations. Look for the irony and absurdity in life.
- **Surround yourself with reminders to laugh.** Choose a computer screensaver that makes you laugh, and frame photos of you and your friends and family having fun.

- **Remember funny things that happen**. If something funny happens to you, write it down so that you remember it to tell others later. Also write down funny jokes you hear, to tell others.
- **Don't dwell on the negative**. Try to avoid negative people and news stories. Many things in our lives are uncontrollable, but we may be able to remove ourselves from hearing about them.
- **Find your inner child**. Try to emulate children: they are often the experts on playing, taking life lightly, and laughing at silly things.
- **Deal with stress**. Stress can be a major impediment to humour and laughter, so try to use strategies to help with your stress levels. Seek professional help if life gets to be too much for you.
- **Don't go a day without laughing**. Make a conscious effort each day that will make you laugh.

EXERCISE 11.4   Have Fun!

Make time for fun activities with your friends and co-workers. This could be karaoke, miniature golf, bowling, or even a games night in your house.

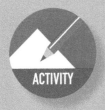

Chapter 11 Activity

These are laughter therapy exercises. Have a go at the ones you feel comfortable with!

Fake laugh	All you need to do for this exercise is laugh, either real or fake, and shrug your shoulders. It is often called the 'I don't know why I'm laughing' exercise and is good for releasing stress.
Have a hearty laugh.	This is a classic yoga laughter exercise. This type of laugh should come from your heart, so it is not a fake laugh. You will need to think of something you can laugh about. Then spread your arms up to the sky, tilt your head back a little, raise your chin – and laugh as heartily as you can. You can bring your arms down if needed.
Cell phone laughter	This is also a classic yoga exercise. Imagine you are holding a cell phone to your ear, listening to someone who something funny at the other end of the line, and laughing at whatever it is they said to you.
Swinging laughter	For this exercise, swing both of your arms gently from side to side while chanting 'ho ho ha ha ha'. This exercise will engage both sides of the brain, the left and right.
Argument laughter	This exercise helps to release stress: voice your discontent and stress through laughing sounds only. No words or other sounds should be heard. You can point fingers and do some actions with your hands.
Jumping frog laughter	To do this exercise, you need to squat down and keep your hands on the floor between your knees. Jump once, and say 'ha'; jump again, and say 'ha ha'; jump again, and say 'ha ha ha'. Continue jumping in fast succession while laughing.
Vowel movement laughter	For this exercise, laugh following these sounds: 'eee eee eee eee! Aye aye aye aye! Ah ah ah ah! Ho ho ho ho! Ooo ooo ooo ooo! Uh uh uh uh!'
Imitation laughter	Start by imitating someone else's voice that you think sounds funny (think of someone on the television or film).
A-O laughter	This exercise should be performed in a group. All members form a wide circle, move forward whilst making a prolonged sound of 'Ae Ae Aeeeee', and then simultaneously wave their hands and burst into laughter once they meet at the centre. After laughing, everyone moves back to their original positions and does the same procedure, but this time using the sound 'Oh Ooooooooo'.

KEY POINTS

- The benefits of laughter
- The physical, mental, and social benefits of humour
- Laughter therapies for stress relief:
  - Humour therapy
  - Clown therapy
  - Meditation with laughter
  - Laughter yoga
  - Laughter clubs
- Caution when using humour
- How to bring more laughter into your life
- How to develop your sense of humour
- Laughter therapy exercises used in healthcare

WEB RESOURCES

Doctor Patch Adams: www.patchadams.org

Top 25 comedy movies: https://www.imdb.com/list/ls0762 33821/

Therapeutic benefits of laughter: https://pubmed.ncbi.nlm. nih.gov/27439375

Laughter is the best medicine: https://www.helpguide.org/ articles/mental-health/laughter-is-the-best-medicine.htm

Managing conflict through humour: https://www.helpguide. org/articles/relationships-communication/managing-conflicts-with-humor.htm

Cultivating happiness: https://www.helpguide.org/articles/ mental-health/cultivating-happiness.htm

Top 10 jokes on Twitter: https//www.independent.co.uk/ voices/top-10-jokes-on-twitter-b2142970.html

Chapter 12

· ·

GUIDED MEDITATION

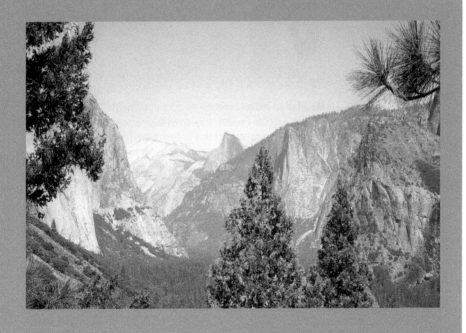

Wellbeing Strategies for Nurses, First Edition. Claire Boyd.
© 2023 John Wiley & Sons Ltd. Published 2023 by John Wiley & Sons Ltd.

LEARNING OUTCOMES

By the end of this chapter, you will have an understanding of meditation and its benefits to health, as well as the different types of meditation, and you will be able to practice both simple and slightly more complex meditation techniques.

First off, meditation does not always involve sitting cross-legged on the nearest mountaintop while 'om-ing' and 'ah-ing' – unless you want to, that is! It can actually be performed anywhere you feel comfortable, such as in the bedroom. Meditation is also not the same thing as hypnotism, so nobody will be made to cluck like a chicken and have no memory of doing so – yes, I really was asked about this during one of my group sessions!

WHAT IS MEDITATION?

Meditation is the practice of concentrated focus on a sound, object, breath, movement, or attention itself to increase awareness of the present moment, reduce stress, promote relaxation, and enhance personal and spiritual growth. You do not always need to be spiritual to enjoy the benefits of meditation – in this chapter, you may wish to just enjoy the experience of the calm and relaxation it brings.

Many meditation practices use **concentration meditation** whereby individuals focus on a single point: breathing, repeating a single word or mantra, staring at a candle flame, or counting beads on a mala.

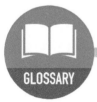

GLOSSARY

Mala
A string of prayer beads.

Meditation is used in the healthcare and education sectors to help reduce anxiety, stress, and pain. It can also benefit individuals requiring a boost of energy.

WHAT ARE THE BENEFITS OF MEDITATION?

Meditation has numerous physiological benefits, one of which is learning to breathe mindfully, using breathing techniques such as **box breathing** and **bellows breathing**.

EXERCISE 12.1   Box Breathing

Sit comfortably in a chair with your feet planted firmly on the ground, shoulder-width apart:

1   Breathe in for four seconds.
2   Hold for four seconds.
3   Exhale for four seconds.
4   Hold for four seconds.
5   Repeat for six cycles.

This technique helps slow the mind by deepening your breathing and induces feelings of calm and serenity, so it is great for treating anxiety and stress.

EXERCISE 12.2   Bellows Breathing

Start with 15 seconds on your first go, working up to one minute. You can increase little by little each time you practise this:

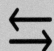

1   Sit tall in a chair with your back straight and your shoulders relaxed.
2   Begin by inhaling and exhaling rapidly through your nose, keeping your mouth closed but relaxed. The in-and-out breaths should be equal in duration but as short and quick as possible. The bellows breathing technique is a noisy breathing exercise.
3   Try for three complete breath cycles per second. As you breathe, you will notice a quick movement of the diaphragm, just like a bellows.

Once this exercise has been completed, you should feel invigorated and alert.

TYPES OF MEDITATION

There are numerous types of meditation, such as:

- Deep breathing exercises
- Relaxation exercises
- Guided imagery
- Progressive relaxation meditation
- Body scan meditation
- Mindfulness meditation

EVIDENCE FOR USING MEDITATION

Amongst the many research studies concerning meditation, researchers from the University of Baltimore showed that meditation could help ease psychological stresses like anxiety, depression, and even pain. It has also been found to help individuals having problems sleeping. These studies have shown that meditation can induce a relaxation response, which can:

- Lower blood pressure
- Improve circulation
- Lower the heart rate
- Slow the respiratory rate
- Help individuals feel less anxious
- Lower blood cortisol levels
- Induce feelings of wellbeing
- Help with stress
- Help individuals obtain deeper levels of relaxation

STUDENT TIP

I read and learn the meditation exercises and then practice them in peace and quiet by myself, although some of my friends record the script on their phone and follow the instructions.

MEDITATION FOR BEGINNERS

Meditation may be difficult at the start, but the more you practise it, the better you will become. A good exercise for the beginner is the following focus meditation, which can be performed anywhere, even during a lunch break.

EXERCISE 12.3   Focus Meditation 1

1   Sit or lie comfortably.
2   Close your eyes.
3   Make no effort to control your breath; simply breathe naturally.
4   Now focus all your attention on your breath.
5   Notice the movement of your body as you breathe.
6   If your mind wanders, return your focus back to your breath.
7   Continue for two to three minutes to start, and then try for longer periods.

Another good meditation exercise when you are a beginner practising this technique is to focus all your attention on an object such as a candle flame or flower. The next exercise focuses on a red rose.

EXERCISE 12.4   Focus Meditation 2

1   Obtain a red rose, sit comfortably, and stare at it for some moments.
2   Imagine yourself touching it and feeling its velvety texture.
3   Pay attention to any lines or creases in the petals.
4   Look at the stem and any leaves.
5   Immerse yourself in the colour red.
6   Imagine the rich, heady perfume of the rose.
7   Continue looking at the beauty of the rose.

During my sessions, I bring in flowers from my garden, so any flower will do for this exercise.

As you can see from this exercise, you may use your imagination when meditating. Scientific research has shown that thoughts produce the same mental responses as actions. Although we will look at visualisation and visiting a tropical island in Chapter 14, visualisation and meditation can be combined successfully. Note that we will also look at the differences between visualisation and meditation in Chapter 16. But let's use our imagination in the next exercise.

EXERCISE 12.5   Focusing on a White Sandy Beach

1   Sit comfortably, and close your eyes.
2   Begin the box breathing exercise (Exercise 12.1).
3   Then, imagine a tropical island with beautiful palm trees.
4   See the turquoise water and clear blue sky.
5   Hear the sound of the soft waves as they roll onto the shore.
6   Feel the soft sand beneath your feet.
7   Feel the warm breeze against your skin.
8   Smell the salt air.
9   Allow your breath to slow down and match the rolling waves of water.
10 Spend some time taking it all in.

Another easy-to-follow exercise using the imagination is the bonfire meditation, which is good for releasing stress and anxiety.

EXERCISE 12.6   Bonfire Meditation

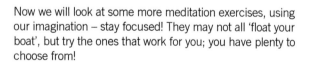

1   Sit down or lie comfortably.
2   Close your eyes.
3   Imagine yourself sitting by a small bonfire.
4   Immerse yourself in the colour of the flames and their warmth.
5   Hear the crackle of the wood as it burns.
6   Notice what is around you, and take the time to sit and silently reflect.

Now we will look at some more meditation exercises, using our imagination – stay focused! They may not all 'float your boat', but try the ones that work for you; you have plenty to choose from!

EXERCISE 12.7   Silver Light

1   Settle into a comfortable position sitting in a chair. Close your eyes. Inhale deeply for the count of 4. Hold for two seconds. Exhale for a count of 4. Repeat this breathing pattern six times, focusing all your attention on your breathing.

2   Place all your attention on your feet. Imagine a bright, silvery white light flowing into both your feet. Feel your feet relaxing. You may feel a slight tingling sensation, but don't worry if you don't, as this will come with practice.

3   Bring the bright light up towards your knees, feeling your legs and knees relax. Imagine bringing the bright light up to your thigh muscles and hips, feeling them relax.

4   The bright light travels up your abdomen, past your stomach and navel area, and towards your heart. All the while, feel the tension leave and the relaxation set in as your muscles relax.

5   As the bright light travels up towards the tip of your heart, feel your chest, shoulders, and neck muscles relax. Release any tension you are holding in your cheeks and forehead.

6   Now bring the bright light down your arms, past the elbows, and out and away through your hands, taking all the tension with it. You may feel a tingling sensation in your hands.

7   Remain in this state of total relaxation, but continue to focus on your breathing. When you are ready, begin to come back to the here and now.

EXERCISE 12.8   The Cinema

1   Settle into a comfortable position sitting in a chair. Close your eyes. Inhale deeply for the count of 4. Hold for two seconds. Exhale for a count of 4. Repeat this breathing pattern six times, focusing all your attention on your breathing.

2   Now imagine you are all alone in a cinema – Vue, Odeon, Cineworld, etc. – you decide whichever has the most comfortable, plush seats.

3   Imagine you are sitting in the middle of the movie theatre in a big, comfortable chair. Your legs and back are fully supported. The large screen is right in front of you. You feel warm, safe, and secure. No one will disturb you.

4   You see the number 20 appear in large, black print on the left-hand side of the screen. Focus on the number 20. As you look at the number, it begins to move slowly to the right until it disappears off the screen. Feel your muscles start to let go, and imagine any tension you are holding gently melting away.

5   The number 19 now appears on the left side of the screen and moves slowly along to the right, disappearing at the edge. You feel more relaxed. Your mind is quiet.

6   Continue counting down, seeing each number travel across the screen from left to right. See the numbers clearly and vividly.

7   18, 17, 16, 15, 14 – you are feeling very relaxed now – 13, 12, 11, 10, 9, 8, 7, 6, . . .

8   Your body feels like it is sinking into the chair. Don't worry if your mind begins to wander; don't fight it, just gently bring your mind back to the movie theatre.

9   See the number 5 slowly make its way across the screen. You are going deeper and deeper.

10 Follow the number 4 as it travels across the screen. Your muscles feel heavy, and you are aware of the silence and stillness around you.

11 Now the number 3 appears on the left side of the screen and drifts slowly to the right. Then the number 2 appears on the left and travels slowly across the screen to the right.

12 The number 1 appears on the left and moves to the right. Your body is completely relaxed. Wait a moment or two, and then get up in your mind's eye and leave the cinema.

Chapter 12 Activity

Floating with the Stars

1   Begin by lying down on a soft, comfortable bed or yoga mat.

2   Close your eyes.

3   Focus on your breathing by going through the diaphragmatic breathing technique (Exercise 4.2).

4   Lie quietly and let your breathing find its own rhythm. Just relax.

5   Imagine you are in a protective transparent bubble. You are safe in this bubble.

6   Feel a sense of lightness. Allow yourself to let go.

7   Feel yourself start to float in the bubble; feel the lightness.

8   The bubble is lifting up beyond the earth's atmosphere and out into the vastness of space. You are safe in the bubble.

9   You look out of the bubble, and everything around you is pitch black, pierced only by the twinkling stars.

10   You are in a beautiful starfield with bright, brilliant points of light.

11   You let your body relax in the enjoyment of floating with the stars.

Leave a long pause.

12   The universe is vast, endless. Continue to relax in this floating sensation amongst the stars.

13   You are peaceful and safe in your bubble, floating amongst the diamond-like stars.

14   You now tune your awareness back into your body.

15   Feeling the weight of gravity once again, your bubble slowly and gently travels back down to earth.

16   Feel the earth's atmosphere as you float down into the room you are in.

17   Your bubble disappears as your body feels the surface you are lying on.

18   Enjoy the magnificent feeling you still retain – the feeling of being one with the universe, floating amongst the stars. That feeling does not leave you.

19   Begin to wiggle your toes and fingers.

20   Roll your shoulders.

21   Stretch your body.

22   Slowly open your eyes, and come back to the here and now

KEY POINTS

- What is meditation?
- What are the benefits of meditation?
- Types of meditation
- Evidence for using meditation
- Meditation for beginners
- Focus meditation
- Meditation using imagination/visualisation

WEB RESOURCES

Meditation exercises: https://www.positivepsychology.com/meditation-exercises-activities, https://www.gaiam.com/blogs/discover/meditation-101-techniques-benefits-and-a-beginner-s-how-to, https://www.verywellmind.com/visualization-for-relaxation-2584112

Chapter 13

· · · · · · · · · · · · · · · · · · ·

MINDFULNESS

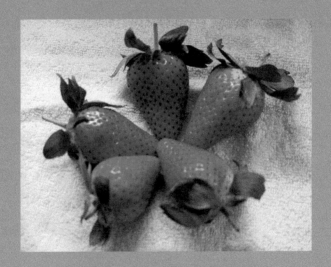

Wellbeing Strategies for Nurses, First Edition. Claire Boyd.
© 2023 John Wiley & Sons Ltd. Published 2023 by John Wiley & Sons Ltd.

LEARNING OUTCOMES

By the end of this chapter, you will have an understanding of mindfulness and the different forms of mindfulness and how they can be used in healthcare for stress relief. You will also be aware of exercises that can be used in mindfulness to focus on the present moment.

Mindfulness is a type of meditation where you focus on being intensely aware of what you are sensing and feeling in the moment. In other words, it's about paying more attention to the present moment to touch base with your thoughts and feelings to improve your wellbeing.

STUDENT TIP

To me, mindfulness is about focus, concentration, and acceptance.

There is no point worrying about what has passed (just let it go) or what the future may hold (as we are not clairvoyant), so just concentrate on what is happening now and try to enjoy it.

One of the stories I tell during my mindfulness sessions is about how we tend to operate on auto-pilot. My husband once offered to drive me to work at the weekend, which I gratefully accepted. I was busy texting in the passenger seat whilst my husband drove the car. The next thing I knew, we had arrived at the local shopping mall, having driven some way right passed the hospital! It does say something about my favourite hobby – shopping! I am sure there are incidences of you also operating on auto-pilot. Just to note, I did get in to work on time for my shift (and broke no traffic laws)!

For those who have practised mindfulness previously, you will no doubt be aware of the famous 'raisin exercise', which we will look at next, but I personally would begin my mindfulness sessions using strawberries or other fruit in season from my garden. This is a great introduction to mindfulness. Of course, you should not take part in this exercise if you are allergic to raisins, or strawberries, or other fruits offered!

EXERCISE 13.1   Raisin Exercise

This exercise is about picking up a raisin (or another piece of fruit) and pretending you have never seen a raisin before in your life:

1   Really look at the raisin and pay careful attention to it.
2   Examine how it looks, paying attention to the wrinkles in the skin.
3   How does it feel between your fingers – soft and lumpy?
4   Gently squeeze it, and see how the skin responds to this manipulation.
5   Smell it – does it smell fruity?
6   Then put it in your mouth and roll it around before you bite into it.
7   What does it taste like?

This exercise is about bringing the mind back to the present and seeing what is right in front of you. We may see raisins frequently, but we do not take the time to notice them.

MINDFULNESS TAKES MANY FORMS

Mindfulness sessions usually begin with some mindful breathing, which we practised in Chapter 4, and may also be combined with guided meditation and the use of imagery and visualisation – taking us to places we can only imagine.

Other examples of mindfulness in action include:

Mindful eating – Paying attention to the taste, sight, and textures of what we are eating.
Mindful moving, walking, or running – Paying attention to the sights and sounds around us and, whilst exercising, how our body feels.
Body scan – Moving our attention slowly through different parts of the body, as we will see in the next section.
Mindful colouring and drawing – We will look at this in Chapter 15.
Mindful meditation – Such as stillness, which we will look at in Chapter 16.

BODY-SCAN MINDFULNESS

The mindfulness body-scan meditation is used at the start of many other relaxation exercises and involves focusing on **feeling** your physical body. During the scanning process, you search for sensations in the body such as tension, strain, or pain, thereby strengthening your connection with your physical self and boosting your physical and mental wellness by anticipating and addressing stress-based physical discomfort.

The body-scanning technique helps you become more aware of how you are feeling at any given moment. When we are stressed, we carry excess muscle tension, which exacerbates muscle pain, headaches, and fatigue; by scanning the body, we can prevent the build-up of this tension and pressure by helping the body progressively relax. It is also thought to reduce the physiological tension caused by thoughts that tend to provoke anxiety.

Scientific research on the practice of body scanning is limited but does show that it may lead some people to experience the benefits associated with mindfulness practices in general, such as:

- Better sleep quality
- Decrease in symptoms of anxiety, depression, and stress
- Management of chronic pain
- Decrease in mental health symptoms associated with chronic pain
- Boost in self-control

There is no hard-and-fast rule as to how long the body-scanning exercise should take; you may wish to spend five minutes or an hour, depending on how much time you have to spare. I would recommend, however, that it is good to spend 15–20 minutes on body scanning.

EXERCISE 13.2   Body Scanning

1   Settle into a comfortable position, sitting in a chair. Close your eyes. Inhale deeply for the count of 4. Hold for two seconds. Exhale for a count of 4. Repeat this breathing pattern six times, focusing all your attention on your breathing.
2   Tune in to and pay attention to any sensations you may feel around your body, like pain, muscle ache, or discomfort. You may notice sensations like tingling.
3   Take another deep breath in through your nose, exhaling through your mouth, releasing any uncomfortable sensation you may feel. Allow this area of your body to release, loosen up, and soften.

4   Work your way up the body, paying attention to how you feel as you focus on your legs, hips, back, stomach, chest, neck and shoulders, arms and hands, and finally face and head.
5   When you have finished scanning, lie still for a moment or two. And when you are ready, go about your day.

MINDFULNESS AIMS TO HELP

Like all the strategies for stress relief, you do not have to be spiritual to benefit from mindfulness. It aims to help individuals:

* Become more self-aware
* Feel calmer and less stressed
* Feel more able to choose how to respond to thoughts and feelings
* Cope with difficult or unhelpful thoughts
* Be kinder to yourself

SCIENTIFIC EVIDENCE FOR USING MINDFULNESS

Studies have shown that practising mindfulness can help to manage common mental health problems, such as:

* Depression
* Anxiety
* Panic attacks
* Stress

There is also some evidence that mindfulness can help with more complex mental health conditions, but more research is needed.

HOW TO PRACTICE MINDFULNESS

To get more out of mindfulness exercises, there are some practical things you can do to help improve your experience:

Set a regular time to practice. Regular, short periods of mindfulness can work better than occasional long ones, so try to practice regularly. If you struggle to find time, try choosing one or two things you already do daily and then do them mindfully: for example, eating an apple or brushing your teeth.

Make yourself comfortable. Some people enjoy doing their mindful exercises outside in nature, but others may prefer to practise mindfulness in the comfort of their own homes – somewhere safe. Find what works for you.

Don't worry if you are doing it right. You may find it strange to practise some of these mindfulness exercises, but don't worry if you are doing the exercises correctly – just enjoy the experience.

Take it slowly. Remember, you are learning a new skill, which may take time to develop.

These next exercises can be performed by individuals or in larger groups. Adapt them to suit; however, the first two exercises are great with a group.

EXERCISE 13.3   The Balloon Game

Balloons are relatively cheap, and all you need for this exercise is one balloon, but you can play with more than one if you want:

1   Sit the group on the floor (or chairs) in a circle.
2   Throw the balloon in the air, and then keep it in the air – avoid letting it touch the ground.

The idea is that you will spend so much time and focus on the balloon(s) that negative thoughts and worries may fade into the background.

EXERCISE 13.4   Cheese Tasting

1   Get a group of friends to each bring one really unique cheese to your house, preferably a kind no one has tasted before.
2   Cut the cheeses into cubes, and sit around tasting them, using the raisin exercise to really explore the taste, smell, texture, etc.

You can supply some crackers and maybe some wine. You can purchase non-dairy cheeses for those who are vegan and non-alcoholic wine for those who don't wish to drink alcohol.

Note: Always check for allergies in all those participating.

EXERCISE 13.5 Happiest Day

Close your eyes, and spend one minute thinking about the happiest day of your life. Try to remember as much about the day as you can.

If you have multiple 'happiest days' and can't choose, try to pick one of the days for different sessions you perform this exercise. This day can be about anything.

MINDFUL JOURNALS

In a mindful journal, you put down on paper where you practice mindfulness in your everyday life. An example of a mindfulness journal can be seen in the next exercise.

EXERCISE 13.6 Mindful Journal

Day	Mindfulness exercise	Mindfulness moments	Mindfulness practised at work/home
Example	Did the body scan exercise when I got home from work. Really noticed the tension in my body and was able to let it go.	Walked to work this morning through the hospital grounds and saw three squirrels – spent a few moments watching them. This made my morning.	Turned off my mobile phone when I went for my break in the staff room so that I would not be distracted from enjoying my break and spending time with my colleagues.
Sunday			
Monday			
Tuesday			
Wednesday			
Thursday			
Friday			
Saturday			

Chapter 13 Activity

ACTIVITY

Chocolate Paradise

This activity is one my colleagues loved during their relaxation sessions: eating chocolate mindfully (dark is best, with a high cocoa content).

1   **Get a small piece of chocolate:** about one square of any chocolate you like.

2   **Relax your body.** Take a few deep breaths, and work on un-tensing your muscles to relax your body. You want to start your chocolate meditation as physically relaxed as possible. Close your eyes.

3   **Smell, gaze, and nibble.** After you smell the chocolate and enjoy the aroma, after you examine the chocolate and really take in how delicious it looks, you can finally take a small bite. Let it sit on your tongue and melt in your mouth. Notice the flavours from the chocolate, and become completely absorbed in what you're experiencing *right now*. Continue your deep breathing, and concentrate on the sensations in your mouth.

4   **Focus on sensations.** As you swallow, focus on how the chocolate feels going down. Notice how your mouth feels empty. Then, as you take a second bite, try to notice how your arm feels as you raise the chocolate to your mouth and how the chocolate feels between your fingers and then in your mouth. Again, focus on the sensations you are feeling in the present moment.

5   **Refocus on the present.** If other thoughts come into your mind during your chocolate meditation, gently refocus your attention on the flavours and sensations associated with the chocolate. The idea is to stay in the present moment as much as you possibly can.

Note: You don't need to consume large quantities of chocolate during this exercise. In fact, if you're doing it carefully, you won't consume much at all. If you are doing this activity in a group, check for allergies before beginning.

KEY POINTS

- What is mindfulness?
- Different forms of mindfulness
- Raisin exercise
- Body-scan mindfulness
- What mindfulness aims to help
- Scientific evidence of using mindfulness
- Mindfulness exercises:
  - The balloon game
  - Cheese tasting
  - Happiest day
  - Mindful journals
  - Chocolate paradise

WEB RESOURCES

- **Mindfulness in healthcare:** https://www.mind.org.uk/information-support/drugs-and-treatments/mindfulness/about-mindfulness, https://www.mind.org.uk/information-support/types-of-mental-health-problems/depression/about-depression, www.mind.org.uk/information-support/types-of-mental-health-problems/anxiety-and-panic-attacks/about-anxiety, www.mind.org.uk/information-support/types-of-mental-health-problems/stress/what-is-stress

Chapter 14

VISUALISATION (GUIDED IMAGERY)

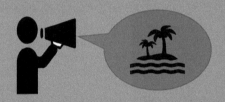

Wellbeing Strategies for Nurses, First Edition. Claire Boyd.

LEARNING OUTCOMES

By the end of this chapter, you will have an understanding of what visualisation is and the benefits of visualisation for health. You will also be able to distinguish between visualisation and meditation, create a relaxing atmosphere for the optimal relaxation experience, and practice visualisation exercises.

Visualisation usually involves closing your eyes in a quiet, calm environment and forming mental visual images of something (or somewhere) you would like to experience: for example, walking on warm sand on a tropical beach.

How many of us have started daydreaming during a lecture or boring meeting, imagining ourselves walking beside a beautiful waterfall! Or is this just me?! If you are prone to daydreaming, like me, we are halfway to practising visualisation: in short, taking a mini-vacation in our mind.

Visualisation helps relax the mind and the body, clearing away the mental chatter of the day, so it is an ideal therapy to use when feeling stressed and anxious. Visualisation practices can evoke all the senses. The first exercise is a classic and can be adapted to all the guided visualisation sessions in Part 3 of this book, such as a walk in the forest. This is a wonderful practice, literally taking just five minutes of your time, and it can be done almost anywhere or any time (obviously not whilst driving a car)! I usually begin my sessions with this exercise. Let's imagine we are on a tropical island.

EXERCISE 14.1   Tropical Island Five-Senses Exercise

This is a quick-fix stress-busting exercise. Spend 50 seconds imagining each item. **(5 MINUTES) Close your eyes.**

Sight
Visualise a palm tree full of lush green leaves. **See it.**

Sound
Think of complete darkness.
Imagine the sound of waves lapping against the shore.
Listen to the seagulls in the sky. **Hear it.**

Smell
Conjure up the smell of fresh, cool, salty sea air. **Smell it.**

Taste
Visualise a lemon. Look at its shape and colour.
Slice it in the middle, and look at the fresh, juicy, glistening flesh. Squeeze it gently, and let the juice drip.
Take the cut end to your mouth, and lick it. **Taste it.**

Touch
Evoke the tactile image of walking barefoot over warm, soft sand on a hot summer's day. **Feel it.**

Kinaesthetic sense (perception of body movement)
Lastly, feel yourself engaged in the activity of climbing a sand dune. **Imagine it.**

EXERCISE 14.2   Countryside Exercise

The Five senses exercise can be adapted to any theme you wish: in this case, the countryside.

Sight
Visualise a delicate, vibrant red poppy swaying in the breeze. **See it.**

Sound
Think of complete darkness.
Imagine the sound of crickets chirping in the warm meadow grass. Listen to the birds in the blue sky. **Hear it.**

Smell
Conjure up the aroma of sweet, newly cut hay on a warm summer's day. **Smell it.**

Taste
Visualise a small, sweet strawberry. Look at the shape and colour. Slice it in the middle, and look at the fresh, juicy, glistening flesh. Squeeze it gently, and let the juice drip.
Take the cut end to your mouth, and lick it. **Taste it.**

Touch
Evoke the tactile image of walking barefoot over newly mown grass on a hot summer's day. **Feel it.**

Kinaesthetic sense
Feel yourself engaged in running through a field of barley. **Imagine it.**

WHAT IS THE DIFFERENCE BETWEEN VISUALISATION AND MEDITATION?

We use meditation to sharpen our focus through **mental exercises**, such as controlled breathing techniques. Visualisation is a technique that allows us to **use our imagination more deeply** to experience joyful experiences, such as walking through a bluebell wood or floating on a cloud. Before you start visualising, it is important to have a relaxed mind. Therefore, meditation is often a prelude to the practice of visualisation. Achieving a meditative state before visualisation helps to enhance self-awareness and focus, keeping your mind alert and enabling you to engage the imagination to visualise the images.

BENEFITS OF VISUALISATION FOR RELAXATION

Visualisation has been used in many areas of healthcare, such as palliative care (imagining healthy cells battling with cancer cells), neurosciences (stroke patients), psychiatry, maternity, cardiac patient, mental health, etc. Evidence shows a positive correlation between visualisation and post-operative pain management, with those using pain management visualisation experiencing less pain and requiring less pharmacological pain management.

Visualisation can also be used in areas such as business (i.e. visualising a big deal coming through) or sports psychology (visualising how you will run the race and win). In short, it is all about creating strong detailed mental images of what you wish to achieve and feeling them. In our case, we are using visualisation to induce the relaxation response to manage stress and anxiety.

Numerous studies have suggested benefits of practising visualisation, including:

- Increases confidence
- Decreases anxiety
- Enhances performance
- Boosts motivation

- Reduces pain
- Relieves stress
- Declutters the mind

DID YOU KNOW?

It is recommended that you read out the scripts on your phone and record them to play back. Visualisation scripts should be read slowly, with plenty of pauses.

Visualisation can be used with other therapies to first relax the body, as in the case of the next exercise.

EXERCISE 14.3   Floating Seaweed

Lie down in a quiet place. Close your eyes. Breathe in deeply once . . . then relax into the rhythm of your natural breathing . . ..

Picture a length of seaweed – rich, dark green, leafy seaweed, floating in the shallows. Air pockets keep it buoyant and allow it to bob up and down. As it floats, it changes shape, drawn this way and that as the currents swirl beneath it . . . pulling it . . . twisting it . . . stretching it . . . bunching it . . ..

Now picture yourself as that piece of seaweed. Notice how limp your body feels . . . your outstretched arms and legs gently swept to and fro . . .. Imagine a wave passing underneath you . . . lifting you up as it rises and lowering you as it dips, but always buoying you up . . .. Feel your body giving in to the movement of the water . . ..

Floating, changing shape, drawn this way and that as the currents swirl beneath you . . . pulling you . . . twisting you . . . stretching you . . . bunching you . . ..

Swirling . . . swirling . . ..

Realize how relaxed you feel. Lie still, and listen to the gently lapping waves all around you. When you are ready, come back to the here and now.

Another simple visualisation exercise is the window technique. When your mind is racing and you can't get to sleep and are feeling stressed about it, try this exercise.

EXERCISE 14.4 Window Technique

Visualise lots of people chatting loudly just outside your open window.
   Instead of getting annoyed and angry, take control.
   Visualise yourself closing the window, and notice how everything has gone quiet.

CREATING A RELAXING ATMOSPHERE

For my group visualisation sessions, I always created the ambience with soothing music and smells. You may wish to look at Chapter 9 to see suggested perfumes for the sessions. During the tropical island session, I would perhaps use the sounds of waves to create the right atmosphere.

Whether you are visualising alone or with a group of friends, it is important to be comfortable and in as noise-free an environment as possible – not always easy in a busy acute hospital. These next exercises are always popular in my group sessions.

EXERCISE 14.5 Floating on a Cloud

Find a relaxed position – lying down is best – and get comfortable. Breathe in and out slowly, and focus on your breathing for a moment or two.

When you are ready, begin to create a picture in your mind. Imagine that you are floating on a soft, fluffy white cloud.

Feel the surface beneath you becoming softer . . . more cloud-like. Feel the cloud rising out of the surface you are on, surrounding you in its protective support . . .. Soon you are floating on just the cloud . . ..

Let it rise a little further, taking you with it . . .. See the walls and ceiling around you disappear as you float into the sunny sky . . . drifting on the cloud.

Feel the cloud beneath you. It is soft but supportive. Feel the cloud supporting your whole body . . ..

Notice each place where your body is touching the cloud. Feel how soft and comfortable the cloud is. It is almost like floating in the air . . ..

Notice how the cloud feels. It might be a bit cool and moist, like fog. Your body is warm . . . very warm and heavy . . . sinking into the cloud. It is a wonderful feeling.

Start to create an image in your mind of where you are. You might be floating just above the ground . . . you can choose to float wherever you like. The sky above you is bright blue, sunny, and inviting. You are warm and comfortable, warmed by the sun's rays shining down peacefully . . ..

There are some other clouds in the sky, floating gently. See them lazily passing by, far above . . ..

Your cloud can float wherever you choose. If you enjoy being high up, you can let your cloud rise into the sky. It is very safe . . . very calming . . . very relaxing. You are so relaxed . . . floating on a cloud . . . supported gently but firmly by your cloud . . . surrounded by the cloud's protective embrace.

See the sights around you as you float on your cloud. Imagine the green grass below, gently blowing in the wind. The grass recedes further away as you rise into the sky . . .. From here, the grass looks like a soft carpet, the wind creating gentle waves in the grass as if it were water . . ..

What else do you see? Perhaps some trees, their leaves whispering in the gentle breeze. You can gaze down on housetops, country roads, and hills . . ..

From this amazing vantage point, you can see around you 360 degrees . . .. The horizon stretches out in a complete circle around you.

Notice in the distance how the hills appear almost blue . . . slightly hazy.

How does it feel to be floating on a cloud? Does it sway gently, like a boat on almost-smooth water? Does it drift in the breeze? Can you feel the movement as you gently float on the cloud? You feel so comfortable . . . so relaxed . . . floating on a cloud . . ..

PAUSE

Continue floating on your cloud, enjoying the sights around you. Up here, the air is very clean.

Look up at the beautiful sky. The clouds that were high above you are much closer now. Some are so close you can almost touch them. Not quite.

Continue floating on a cloud . . . drifting . . . rising even higher if you wish.

The ground below you looks like a patchwork quilt. Green grass . . . golden fields . . . yellow . . . brown. Blue patches of water . . . rivers and lakes.

See the clouds around you. You are even able to look down on some clouds. See the shadows they make on the ground below. Can you see the shadow from your cloud? See how the shadow drifts silently across the ground below . . . .

Relax and luxuriate in this beautiful scene, floating on a cloud. You are so close to another cloud above you that if you reach out, you can touch it. What would it feel like?

You can even rise higher still and pass right through the clouds above. Feel the mist on your cheeks as you rise through the clouds. Around you, it is a glorious white, like fog . . . the sun shines through just enough that the white all around you glows vibrantly.

You rise higher still, suddenly coming through the clouds and into the open, dazzling sunlight shining on your face. The sky above is brilliant blue.

You can look down on the cloud you just passed and see the white, fluffy peaks and valleys of this cloud below. It looks like perfect snow. Looking around below you, it is as if you are above a land of snow. The sun shines brightly.

Lie back on your cloud, floating . . . relaxing . . . floating on a cloud.

Feel the cloud beneath you . . . still supporting you smoothly and comfortably.

Take your cloud wherever you wish . . . higher, lower, side to side . . . drift wherever you want to go.

Enjoy the sights around you as you fly wherever you wish . . . ..

PAUSE

Now it is time to return to your day. Let your cloud take you there . . . .. Feel your cloud flying through the sky, back to where you need to go. Let your cloud lower you down, back towards the ground. Float back to where you were when you started this visualisation. Let the cloud melt with the bed, chair, or whatever surface you are on. Feel the cloud slowly disappear as the real surface becomes more solid beneath you.

Notice your surroundings. Gradually come back to the present. Feel the surface beneath you . . . hear the sounds around you . . . become more and more aware and alert. Continue to rest for a few moments, but open your eyes and look around. See your surroundings.

Wiggle your fingers and toes, feeling your body reawaken. Shrug your shoulders. Move your arms and legs. Turn your head. When you are ready, you can return to your day, feeling refreshed and alert after your journey floating on a cloud.

EXERCISE 14.6   Going Through the Tunnel

Imagine yourself strolling along a very straight flat path. It is a dull, cloudy, drizzly sort of day.

The path leads between two high banks. There is damp grass beneath your feet, and you can see the cloudy sky above.

Somehow you feel heavy; you are aware of a heavy backpack on your shoulders, making your steps heavy and slow. Your back is bent a little to support the weight, and you seem to be looking at the ground in front of you as you trudge along the path, feeling damp, cold, and weighed down.

You glance up and see the entrance to an old railway tunnel; this must be a disused railway line.

You can see a point of light at the other end of the tunnel, so it cannot be too long. You decide to continue on your walk . . . at least you will be out of the drizzle in there.

As you approach the entrance, the tunnel seems very dark, but that small circle of light at the far end is reassuring, so you keep moving forward into the tunnel . . ..

At first it seems very dark . . . you can hardly see, but the floor feels even, and it is easy to walk along. As you do so, all those old doubts about yourself begin to surface in your mind . . . you are aware of your own feelings and those things you wish you hadn't done, and the things you wish you had done in the past . . ..

Just let them come gently to the surface of your mind. The backpack seems to be getting a little lighter as these different doubts and regrets unpack from your inner mind gently and easily.

You keep walking and notice a pool of light on the floor ahead . . ... There must be an air shaft.

As you go through this pool of light, you suddenly remember a happy time when someone enjoyed your company . . . a time when you felt really good about being you.

As you move out of the light into the darkness again, you feel lighter . . .. The backpack is emptying, and you are standing a little straighter now, but the doubts are rising to the surface. The regrets are floating up into your mind again.

The circle of light at the end of the tunnel is getting bigger now, but here is another air shaft, with that shaft of light penetrating the gloom of the tunnel . . ..

Again, as you pass through the light, another good memory of being appreciated for who you are, being praised for something, or being complimented comes to the forefront of your mind.

Now you are back in the gloom, but it doesn't seem as intense as before. It is getting lighter and warmer step by step, and more and more good memories of those who have loved you and events that pleased you come into your mind . . ...

As you get nearer to the end of the tunnel, you notice that the sun must be shining because it looks very bright out there . . . and you find that you feel much lighter, as if you have lost that backpack altogether . . . .. A pleasant warmth is beginning to replace any traces of damp and cold that you felt before.

Eventually, you step out into the bright summer sunshine, smell the aroma of freshly cut grass, and walk with a light tread into the warmth of a bright summer's day, feeling lighter and valuing yourself and the world around you much more.

You notice a stone bench on the grass verge and sit for a while to rest. You realise how lucky you are to be alive – what a wonderful world. Close your eyes and relax in the warm sunbeam whilst relaxing music is playing in the background. When you are ready, come back to the here and now.

Chapter 14 Activity

ACTIVITY

Mountain Visualisation

Lie down or sit comfortably.

Take a few moments just sitting with your eyes closed. Focus on your breathing: breathe in deeply and slowly through your nose, silently counting to 4. Slowly exhale through your mouth, again counting to 4. Try to make your diaphragm rise and fall, but keep your chest and shoulders still.

Whilst breathing in, visualise warm air flowing to all parts of your body. Whilst breathing out, imagine all the tension and stress leaving your body.

When you are ready, imagine it is a warm summer evening. You are walking along the shore of a small mountain lake. The lake is deserted except for a lone fisherman casting from the shore.

The sun is sinking fast behind the silhouette of trees on the far shore, throwing the last rays across the water.

There is a moment of perfect stillness in the silent twilight between day and night, except for the light splash of a fish . . . and the last sweet notes of a bird's evening song.

A full moon has risen, its light reflecting on the still lake. The night is filled with the sweet fragrance of pine, and you feel the worries and concerns of the day slipping away. All is still . . . you are flooded with a warm feeling of contentment and peace.

A moonbeam appears just in front of you amongst some long, soft grass.

You lie down on this soft sweet smelling grass and feel the beauty of the moment . . .. Rest a while.

Now it is time to return to the here and now. Slowly let the image of the mountain lake fade away. Open your eyes and become aware of your surroundings.

Take a few short breaths, and stretch your body.

KEY POINTS

- What is visualisation?
- Differences between visualisation and meditation
- Benefits of visualisation
- Creating a relaxing atmosphere
- Visualisation exercises

WEB RESOURCES

Visualisation: https://synctuition.com/blog/visualizing-health-deep-relaxation

Visualisation health benefits: https://drgiamarson.com/the-benefits-of-visualization

Chapter 15

ARTS AND CRAFTS

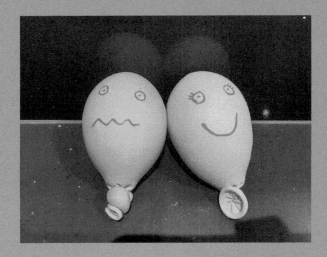

Wellbeing Strategies for Nurses, First Edition. Claire Boyd.
© 2023 John Wiley & Sons Ltd. Published 2023 by John Wiley & Sons Ltd.

LEARNING OUTCOMES

By the end of this chapter, you will have an understanding of how arts and crafts can be used effectively as part of a treatment program for those experiencing stress and anxiety. Many examples of crafting ideas will be shown.

I am pretty sure we have all heard about art therapy, as this has long been an established strategy used in mental health and wellbeing. I am also pretty sure that you know/have viewed some of Van Gogh's masterpieces – just one being his painting of bright yellow sunflowers. You have probably also seen Edvard Munch's 'The Scream'. Both these painters suffered from mental illness, including depression, and found that expressing their feelings on canvas soothed their symptoms somewhat.

Art therapy does not have to consist of painting, as those of you in the mental health or learning disabilities sector know, as other art therapy exercises may be used, such as sculpting, acting, dancing – in short, anything creative you enjoy. Although art therapy can help with anxiety, depression and depressive symptoms, panic attacks, and post traumatic stress disorder (PTSD), to name just a few, you don't have to have mental health issues to enjoy the benefits of art therapy.

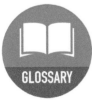

GLOSSARY

PTSD
Post traumatic stress disorder. A mental health condition that develops following a traumatic event.

ART THERAPY TO ALLEVIATE STRESS

Art therapy has been found to be effective in the treatment of stress for the following reasons:

- Acts as a form of self-care when we forget to care for ourselves – slows the frantic pace.
- Enables a 'state of flow', which psychologists describe as being so engrossed in an activity that a state similar to meditation may be achieved.
- Utilises distraction to take your mind off whatever is stressing you (for a short while, at least).

Note: You may have wondered why so many stress-relief activities in this book contain practical tasks – now all will be explained!

Following are 12 art therapy activities that you may wish to consider to help reduce your stress.

Colouring Books for Adults

These books can be purchased relatively cheaply and, with a couple of coloured pencils, can produce a state of calm. You can also print off free designs from the internet, or you can sketch a simple rainbow yourself to colour.

EXERCISE 15.1   Colour a Rainbow

Draw a rainbow and colour it – red, orange, yellow, green, blue, indigo, and violet. Appendix B has a ready-made rainbow for you to colour in.

DID YOU KNOW?

Here is how to remember the colours of the rainbow: Richard Of York Gave Battle In Vain.

R = Red
O = Orange

Y = Yellow
G = Green
 = Blue
I = Indigo
V = Violet

For goodness sake, Richard, it's supposed to relieve your stress! It doesn't matter if you colour outside of the lines!

Create Mandalas

Carl Jung was one of the original proponents of using mandalas as a strategy for stress relief, and they have been used in art therapy for decades. **Mandalas** are geometric circular designs (circles within circles) that often include intricate patterns and symbols in the gaps. These can then be coloured however you like. Mandalas are thought to bring feelings of peace and tranquillity, producing a sense of calmness in a state similar to meditation.

EXERCISE 15.2   Draw a Mandala

Create your own Mandala.

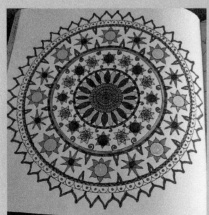

DID YOU KNOW?

Mandala means 'circle' in Sanskrit. Mandalas are sacred symbols used for meditation, prayer, healing, relaxation, and art therapy.

Mindless Doodles

Grab a pencil, and scribble mindlessly – just go with the flow. There is not a lot of specific research on the stress-relieving effects of random doodles, but there is enough information on 'art' in general and its stress-relieving effects to suggest that doodling certainly can't harm. Buy an inexpensive exercise book, and doodle away. Doodling is said to encourage mindfulness.

EXERCISE 15.3   Draw Some Doodles

Get a fresh piece of paper, and fill it with mindless doodles.

Place Stars in the Night Sky

For this exercise, you will need a dark piece of paper (blue or black works well). Draw stars using a white or yellow pencil. With each star you paint, think about all the blessings you have in your life.

EXERCISE 15.4   Draw Stars

Draw stars on paper, and for each star, reflect on a blessing in your life.

Listen to Meditative or Relaxing Music

Music is said to be food for the soul. Music as a therapy, according to a 2020 study, can:

- Lower your heart rate and cortisol levels
- Release endorphins and improve your sense of wellbeing

- Distract you, thereby reducing your physical and emotional stress levels
- Reduce stress-related symptoms, whether used in a clinical environment or in daily life

Other studies indicate that music can also:

- Be beneficial in mental health treatments
- Reduce burn-out
- Help you fall asleep
- Reduce depression
- Reduce anxiety
- Improve quality of life in Alzheimer's disease
- Help relieve both chronic and post-operative pain

Music does not have to be tuneful – many prefer to listen to nature sounds, such as waves rolling on a beach, rain, thunder etc., which can be accessed on free internet sites. So, when you have a free moment, lie on your bed, close the door, and put on a relaxation download – how about the sound of the waves?

EXERCISE 15.5   Listen to Soothing Sounds

Take some time out to listen to soothing music, the sound of waves on a tropical beach, or, if you prefer, the sound of wind and rain or perhaps a momentous thunderstorm.

DID YOU KNOW?

Musicians, neuroscience researchers, and music therapists claim to have created the most relaxing piece of music ever! Neuroscientists in a study found that 65% of participants listening to the tune had a reduction in overall anxiety. The music is said to stir your soul and calm your nervous system (https://www.inc.com/melanie-curtin/neuroscience-says-listening-to-this-one-song-reduces-anxiety-by-up-to-65-percent.html). The song is called 'Weightless'. What do you think?.

Prepare a Song List

We know that music can create a feeling of peace and calm when we play our favourite tunes. The type of music you listen to may have different effects on your mood:

- Classical music is associated with a soothing, calming effect.
- Rap music can be inspiring and motivating when you are experiencing a low mood or dealing with a difficult life situation.
- Heavy metal music can enhance identity development and help you process negative emotions.

When do we get the best benefit from listening to our music?

- **When getting up** – This helps to start the day positively. Classical music can help wake you up in the morning whilst keeping us calm and focused.
- **When going to work** – This helps you arrive less stressed and ready to start the day.
- **When coming home from work** – This can help you wind down from the trials and tribulations of the day and take your mind off work.
- **Before bed** – Playing music as you drift off can take your mind off what is stressing you. Music can help slow down your breathing and soothe the mind.

EXERCISE 15.6   Listen to Favorite Songs

Prepare your own personal song list, and enjoy!

DID YOU KNOW?

As we listen to music, simply put:

1   Music sound waves move through our ears as vibrations.
2   The inner ear translates these vibrations into electrical signals.

3   Neurons transmit these signals to certain areas of the cerebral
    cortex in the brain.
4   Dedicated regions of the brain detect the different elements of
    the signals (such as tone, pitch, and rhythm).
5   The brain puts together all of this information so that you can
    sense the musical experience.

Music can influence our emotions and bodily systems, which is why
scientists are so interested in studying music and its effects.

Photograph Nature or Happy Events

In Chapter 6, we looked at the benefits of nature for our
wellbeing. When going for a walk, take time to actually look
around and take some photographs. You don't need an
expensive, technical camera to take the photo; a phone will
do. Another calming exercise is to look through happy
photos, perhaps of an enjoyable day, of your loved ones, or
of a family wedding. Looking through photos of loved ones
and happier times has been proven to help reduce stress
and decrease anxiety.

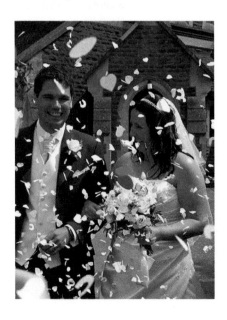

EXERCISE 15.7   Look at Photos

Look through some photos on your phone or in a photo album of a happy event, perhaps a wedding or a holiday.

Dance Like No One Is Watching

Put on your favourite song, and start moving and grooving, releasing all those endorphins. When the body feels good, the mind does, too. By dancing, you are releasing not just your frustrations and anger but also your stress and worries with every move you make. Dancing can:

- Improve us mood and focus
- Provide a creative outlet to express your emotions
- Soothe muscles and arching joints
- Improve physical health:
  - ✓ Improves heart and lung health
  - ✓ Increases stamina
  - ✓ Improves balance and coordination
  - ✓ Improves self-confidence and self-esteem
  - ✓ Improves mental strength and performance

EXERCISE 15.8   Dance!

Clear a space in a room in your home, put on some music, and dance your heart out (not literally – that would not be good, as we need our hearts)!

Make a Stress Ball

Chapter 5 showed a picture of a stress ball with two aliens popping out when the ball is squeezed! Stress balls are malleable toys that are squeezed in the hand and manipulated by the fingers to relieve stress. They can also be used to exercise hand muscles during rehabilitation. Stress balls act as a distraction from the issues causing you stress. You can make your own stress ball.

EXERCISE 15.9   Make a Stress Ball

Make your own stress ball! All you need is a balloon, some play dough (you can also use beans or flour – self-raising or plain, it doesn't matter!), and a permanent marker pen.

Roll the play dough into sausage shapes, get someone to hold open the neck of the balloon, and stuff the play dough into the balloon (Figure 15.1). Keep squeezing play dough into the balloon until it is filled enough, and tie a knot in the balloon (Figure 15.2). Lastly, draw a face on the balloon (Figure 15.3).

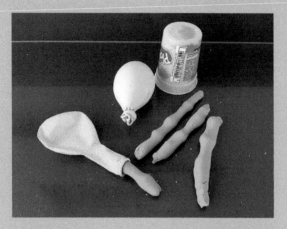

Figure 15.1   Filling balloon.

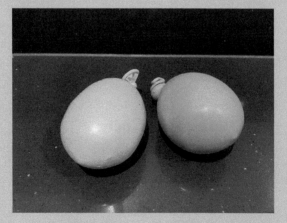

Figure 15.2   Tying the Stress Ball.

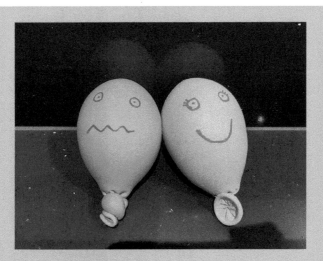

Figure 15.3 Completed stress ball.

Gardening for Stress Relief

A recent study asked subjects to perform a stressful task and then perform either 30 minutes of reading or 30 minutes of gardening. Whilst both groups experienced a decrease in stress, the gardeners experienced a significantly greater decline in stress (as measured by the stress hormone in saliva – cortisol) as well as a full restoration of positive mood. You can create a riot of colours, a beautiful piece of art, in your garden; or if you don't have much money to spend, a pot or two of herbs grown from seed on your windowsill can have the added benefit of being tasty! Gardening can be beneficial to our health:

- Getting out in the sunlight can improve our mood.
- Getting in touch with nature can help us become removed from the stressors in our life.
- Creating beauty is always good for wellbeing.

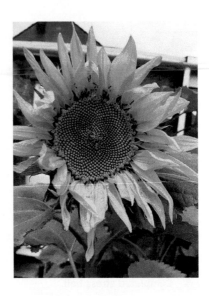

EXERCISE 15.10   Grow Some Plants

Buy a few pots, and fill them with compost. You can go to a high street store where they sell everything for £1, so this does not have to be expensive. Sprinkle on some seeds, water them, and sit back and watch your plants grow. Don't forget to talk to them! Isn't nature wonderful?

Build Something from LEGO Bricks

These coloured Danish bricks can provide relief from stress and anxiety. According to research, 91% of adults find play helpful in managing stress and anxiety because it:

- **Boosts creativity** – By creating defined structures, you can boost many functions in your brain's frontal cortex. When you are stressed, the prefrontal cortex (PFC) of your brain is impaired by catecholamine, hindering your creative juices and thinking abilities.
- **Is a fun activity** – Having regular fun in your life can help boost your mood. Fun activities are a source of eustress for the body, evoking a sense of excitement – the feeling you get from achieving a goal in life.

DID YOU KNOW?

Lots of celebrities like to build with LEGO bricks to aid their relaxation: David Beckham, Ed Sheeran, Britney Spears, and Serena Williams, to name but a few.

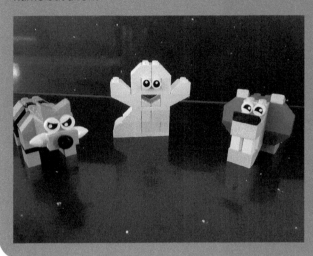

EXERCISE 15.11   Build With LEGO Bricks

Buy a small LEGO model, follow the instructions, and enjoy building. If you have more money to spend, you can buy beautiful LEGO Bonsai models – and they won't die due to lack of water or sunshine!! You could also 'borrow' bricks from family or friends and create something of your own design.

Create a Snowflake from Paper

Making a paper snowflake is a distraction from your stress, as you become engaged in concentrating on the task at hand. To make a snowflake, all you need is a piece of paper and some scissors:

1   Fold a square piece of paper into a triangle (you can use a piece of A4 paper and just cut off the excess to make a square).
2   Fold the triangle in half again to make a smaller triangle.
3   Fold the Right -Hand side of the triangle so that you are folding it into thirds.
4   Repeat the fold as you did for step three, this time on the other side.
5   Use scissors to cut straight across the top, leaving you with a thin, folded triangle.
6   Now for the fun bit! Cut any shape into the folded snowflake, being careful not to make any cuts that go all the way across (this will break your snowflake).
7   When you are happy with your shapes, unfold the paper to reveal your beautiful snowflake design.

EXERCISE 15.12   Cut Snowflakes

Make half a dozen snowflakes, and stick them to your window. Watch as the light peeps through your design, perhaps creating patterns in your room.

CRAFTING AS STRESS RELIEF

Whilst it is not technically art therapy, crafting has long been used in the pursuit of wellness.

GLOSSARY

Crafting
The activity or hobby of making decorative articles by hand. A form of self-expression.

Crafting projects can help the brain send signals to the body that everything is well. Blood pressure and tension are reduced, resulting in a sense of wellbeing. Crafting can mean many different things to many different people, but it usually involves something like this:

- Jewellery making
- Knitting
- Crocheting
- Cake decorating
- Pottery
- Paper crafts
- Embroidery
- Photography
- Quilting
- Papier-mâché
- Sewing
- Scrapbooking

To name just a few!

Neuroscientists explain why crafting is good for mental health: a study conducted with 3545 knitters found that they felt calmer, happier, less sad, less anxious, and more confident. Those who knitted more frequently reported more mental and emotional relief than those who did it less frequently. Therefore, knitting was found to positively impact the mind, health, and wellbeing. It was thought that knitting achieved a meditative state of mind.

Some hospital trusts run knitting groups for staff to attend, known as 'knit and natter' groups, making a social event of the craft. The next exercise is a knitting pattern for a 'twiddle muff' used for care of elderly patients and designed for the less expert knitter to make. Twiddle muffs can benefit those using them and the crafter knitting them.

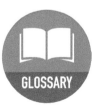

GLOSSARY

Twiddle muff

A twiddle muff is like a hand muff, made with a variety of wool offcuts as well as twiddly bits sewn on both the inside and the outside. Twiddle muffs can be used for both sensory activities and anxiety-relieving activities with sufferers of autism and dementia. Dementia sufferers can become stressed in the unfamiliar surroundings of a hospital or nursing home, which can lead to fiddling with medical equipment such as IV lines, urine catheter bags, dressings, etc. A twiddle muff can keep busy fingers occupied.

EXERCISE 15.13   Make a Twiddle Muff

It is usual to put the patient's name on the twiddle muff so that it will not be used by anyone else (for infection-control purposes), and all attachments should be secured well so that they cannot be pulled off.

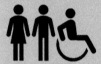

What you need:

- 8 mm knitting needles
- Oddments of leftover chunky wool
- Darning needle
- Buttons, beads, etc. for decoration

Cuff: Cast on 45 stitches. Work in stocking stitch (knit a line, purl a line) for 11 inches.

Muff body: Continue in stocking stitch but use oddments of various textures, such as ribbon, mohair, aran, etc., until the work measures 23 inches. Cast off loosely.

Finishing: Neatly join the long sides together using edge-to-edge stitching (with the knit side facing out). Turn inside out and push the one-colour cuff up inside the muff body. Sew the two ends together, again using a neat edge-to-edge stitch.

Decoration: Decorate the muff inside and out with beads, knitted flowers, buttons, etc.

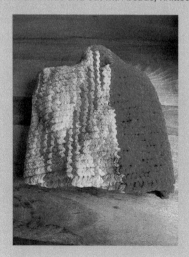

For those at the other end of the spectrum, hats and mittens can be made for premature babies.

EXERCISE 15.14   Make a Preemie Hat

What you need:

- 8 mm knitting needles
- 1 ball of double knit baby wool

Cast on 56 stitches loosely.

Ribbing:

1   Alternate knit 2 stitches, purl 2 stitches to end
2   Next row: purl 2 stitches, knit 2 stitches to end
3   Repeat rows 1 and 2 four more times

Main body:

1   Knit one row
2   Purl one row
3   Repeat alternating for 16 rows

Shaping the crown:

1   Knit 6 stitches, then knit 2 stitches together (i.e. drop one stitch), repeat to end
2   Next row purl entire row
3   Knit 5 stitches, then knit two together, repeat to end
4   Purl entire row
5   Knit 4 stitches, then knit two together, repeat to end
6   Purl entire row
7   Knit 3 stitches, then knit two together, repeat to end
8   Purl entire row
9   Knit 2 stitches, then knit two together, repeat to end
10 Purl entire row

Completing:

1   Cut yarn, leaving sufficient length to sew up the hat
2   Thread end of yarn through remaining stitches on needle
3   Draw tightly, and fasten off securely
4   Sew up edges to form hat

Note: You can use a different colour for the crown section, if you wish.

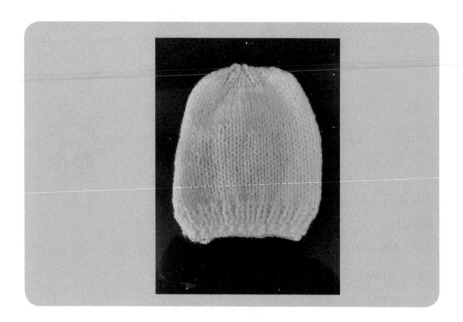

PUZZLES

Modern jigsaw puzzles have been around since 1767 and crossword puzzles in newspapers since 1913. The types and varieties of puzzles are almost endless: jigsaw puzzles, crosswords, wordsearches, Rubix cubes, Tetris, etc. The following are seven specific ways that puzzles are good for the brain:

1   **Puzzles exercise both sides of the brain.** The left hemisphere of the brain controls analytic and logical thinking, and the right hemisphere controls creativity. When you are working on a puzzle, you are engaging both sides and giving your brain a real mental workout.
2   **Puzzles improve your memory.** Working on puzzles reinforces the connections between the brain cells. We use memory in the process of completing a jigsaw puzzle when we remember shapes, sizes, and pieces and visualise where they fit in.
3   **Puzzles improve our problem-solving skills.** The ability to solve problems and think critically is useful in almost any life situation, and puzzles help us develop these skills.

4   **Puzzles improve visual and spatial reasoning.** We need to be able to look at individual parts of a jigsaw puzzle or available spaces in a crossword puzzle and work out how to fit the pieces or words into their space. If done regularly, this is shown to improve these visual and spatial reasoning skills.

5   **Puzzles enhance our mood.** Puzzles increase the production of dopamine – the neurotransmitter that regulates mood, memory, and concentration. Dopamine is released with every success as we solve the puzzle.

6   **Puzzles lower our stress levels.** Puzzles invigorate our brains, but they are also very relaxing. Whilst we are concentrating on how to solve the puzzle, our minds are on only one task, which encourages our brains to go into a meditative state. This leads to a better mindset and better stress coping skills.

7   **Puzzles can improve our IQ score.** Puzzles can improve our memory, concentration, vocabulary, and reasoning skills. Studies have shown that doing puzzles for at least 25 minutes a day can boost your IQ by 4 points.

EXERCISE 15.15   Play Wellness Bingo

Have a game of wellness bingo, found in Appendix D. Cross off as many squares as you can in a one-month time period.

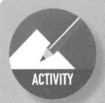

Chapter 15 Activity

Just for a bit of fun, have a go at finding the words in this word search. Answers can be found in the Answers to Activities.

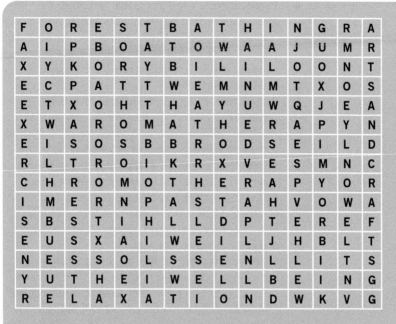

F	O	R	E	S	T	B	A	T	H	I	N	G	R	A
A	I	P	B	O	A	T	O	W	A	A	J	U	M	R
X	Y	K	O	R	Y	B	I	L	I	L	O	O	N	T
E	C	P	A	T	T	W	E	M	N	M	T	X	O	S
E	T	X	O	H	T	H	A	Y	U	W	Q	J	E	A
X	W	A	R	O	M	A	T	H	E	R	A	P	Y	N
E	I	S	O	S	B	B	R	O	D	S	E	I	L	D
R	L	T	R	O	I	K	R	X	V	E	S	M	N	C
C	H	R	O	M	O	T	H	E	R	A	P	Y	O	R
I	M	E	R	N	P	A	S	T	A	H	V	O	W	A
S	B	S	T	I	H	L	L	D	P	T	E	R	E	F
E	U	S	X	A	I	W	E	I	L	J	H	B	L	T
N	E	S	S	O	L	S	S	E	N	L	L	I	T	S
Y	U	T	H	E	I	W	E	L	L	B	E	I	N	G
R	E	L	A	X	A	T	I	O	N	D	W	K	V	G

These 14 words are hidden in the grid.

- Stress
- Breathing
- Biophilia
- Exercise
- Chromotheapy
- Aromatherapy
- Humour
- Stillness
- Relaxation
- Orthosomnia
- Forest bathing
- Fika
- Arts and craft
- Wellbeing

KEY POINTS

Art therapy to alleviate stress:

- Colouring books for adults
- Creating mandalas
- Mindless doodling
- Making stars
- Listening to relaxing music
- Preparing song lists
- Photographing nature/happy events
- Dancing
- Making stress balls
- Gardening
- Building with LEGO bricks
- Making snowflakes

Crafting as stress relief:

- Knitting

Crosswords/wordsearches/puzzles

WEB RESOURCES

Art therapy for stress relief: https://www.verywellmind.com/art-activities-for-stress-relief-3144589

Arts and crafts for stress relief: https://www.psychreg.org/arts-crafts-relieving-stress

Calming crafts: https://ohclary.com/calming-crafts-for-adults

Relaxing crafts: https://www.carlaschauer.com/relaxing-crafts-activities-reduce-anxiety/

Puzzles: https://www.goodnet.org/articles/7-surprising-ways-puzzles-are-good-for-your-brain

Chapter 16

STILLNESS

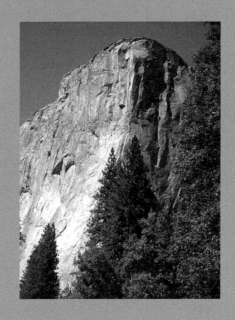

LEARNING OUTCOMES

By the end of this chapter, you will have an understanding of the health principle of stillness, how to practice stillness, the benefits of stillness, and how stillness can help connect you with your senses. You will also be able to perform stillness exercises.

Stillness is a form of meditation that uses relaxation of the body to quiet and calm the mind. It is an efficient relaxation technique used to release physical tension, especially for those experiencing anxiety and/or insomnia.

Stillness meditation is a medical-based therapy that is about helping us to experience our own calm, our own silence, and our own stillness. By spending time doing nothing, we are giving our brain some much-needed rest and relaxation in our awake hours.

PRACTISING STILLNESS

In today's world, so much is going on around us that we may find it difficult to experience any quiet time. Noise can be both inside and outside our brains. After working a busy shift, I could still hear the 'BING, BING BONG' of the volumetric pumps in my head and worried whether I had told my colleagues everything they needed to know during handover. In short, it could be very hard to 'turn off' when work finished. This is where the principle of stillness comes into its own, creating an intention of stillness to soothe our nervous system and replenish our frazzled minds.

Those who practice stillness regularly state that it can be achieved even when chaos swirls all around us – even in places such as shopping malls and airports!

Stillness can take many forms, from the practice of meditation to simply taking the time to sit outside in silence for a few moments each day, doing nothing but breathing. If we experience stress during a difficult shift at work and then more stress is piled on, this is where stillness comes into its own – as a form of self-care. Take some time out: retreat to a quiet place, close the door, and leave what happened in the past. Enjoy the calm for a few moments and then come back to the job, hopefully better able to deal with things.

BENEFITS OF PRACTISING STILLNESS

Stillness gives us the time and space to self-reflect, allowing us to hear our own thoughts. It soothes the nervous system and, used in conjunction with concentrating on our breathing, induces the parasympathetic system and slows the heart rate. Mental chatter dials down, and we feel refreshed. Some of the benefits of practising stillness include:

- **Helps with feelings of stress** – Being in stillness reduces responses in the parasympathetic system: our fight-or-flight response. It increases the responses in the sympathetic system: our rest-and-relaxation response. Stillness can help to calm the mind, helping you feel more at peace and less stressed.
- **Helps you cope with stressful situations** – The peace that comes from practising stillness can help you deal with difficult situations. You may not be able to change your difficult situation, but practising stillness may give you clarity, helping you to respond to the situation differently.
- **Anchors you to the present** – Anxiety and stress often involve us looking to the future – what could go wrong. Stillness anchors you to the present moment so that you can deal with what is happening now and not what might happen in the future.
- **Increases listening skills** – As you learn to be present, you may stop wanting to talk and instead learn to actually hear what others are saying, meaning you may respond more effectively and empathetically.
- **Lets you hear your intuition** – Around the chaos of life, we may have many voices telling us what to do, how to be, what to say, etc. In stillness, we learn to silence these voices, tapping into our intuition.
- **Improves sleep** – The generally relaxed state achieved in stillness can help us fall asleep more easily, leading to a more restful night's sleep. Stillness can also help you fall back to sleep faster if you wake up in the middle of the night.

STUDENT TIP

Stillness, or the state of doing nothing, is actually crucial for our wellbeing. If you don't take 'time-outs', you are more likely to reach your saturation point and experience the harmful effects of stress.

HOW TO PRACTICE STILLNESS

As with any relaxation technique, the more you practice stillness, the better at it you will become. Following are some tips to enable you to experience one of my favourite techniques, which can be performed anywhere, even whilst having a warm bubble bath:

- **Breathe**. Start by taking slow, deep breaths to induce the parasympathetic nervous system to slow your heart rate.
- **Practice when you need it**. Even during a work shift, go into the toilet where you will not be disturbed, and take a few minutes for yourself.
- **Schedule stillness**. At the end of your working day, schedule some stillness time to recharge your batteries.
- **Find a favourite spot**. Even though you can create stillness anywhere, start by choosing a favourite spot. This spot could be outdoors, such as a park or bench, or in your own home – somewhere you can have complete silence.
- **Listen to soft music**. Some people do not like complete silence, so they prefer to have soft, slow music in the background.
- **Repeat calming phrases**. Some people like to repeat calming phrases, such as 'I am calm and still'.

As a very simple stillness exercise, we can start with just using our imagination to picture ourselves somewhere serene and away from the chaotic moment – imagination can transport us anywhere where we feel calm. We may also choose somewhere we have already been and use our memories to evoke the pictures in our mind.

EXERCISE 16.1 Our Special Place

Think of somewhere relaxing and peaceful: This can be a memory of somewhere you have already been or a place you have just imagined.

Close your eyes and think about the details of this place.

Take a moment to think about what it looks like. What are the colours and shapes that you see?

Can you hear any sounds? Is it warm or cold?

Let your mind drift and your body relax.

FAIRY CHAIR

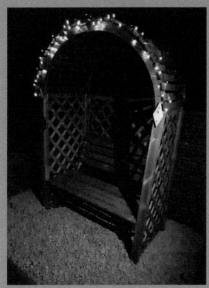

One of my favourite places to practice stillness is on the fairy chair in my garden. Sometimes I like to sit, wrapped in comfy blankets, with one of my favourite people in the world: my grandson. We just cuddle and look up into the starry night sky. It gives us a perspective of our place in the universe.

CONNECTING WITH YOUR SENSES

Bringing in the five senses is a good way of evoking stillness to ground yourself when you are feeling stressed or over-whelmed. This next exercise can be performed anywhere, at home or at work, and takes very little time to perform to achieve the stillness you want.

EXERCISE 16.2   Five Senses Stillness

Stop and just stand where you are:

LOOK – Look around you, and notice five things you can see. Spend a moment or two looking at each item. This could be a pen, the paint on the wall, what you are wearing, rain or sunshine out the window, or your feet. Name these in your head or out loud, but take your time.

TOUCH – Name four things you can touch or feel around you. Spend a moment or two feeling them. This could be your hair, the ground under your feet, the heat or cool or environment around you, or an item in your vicinity.

HEAR – Name three things you can hear around you. It could be the chatter of colleagues, sounds outside, or your breathing.

SMELL – Name two things you can smell around you. It does not have to be a strong smell. Perhaps take a short walk around to find something (in the hospital environment, this should not be too hard!).

TASTE – Name one thing you can taste at the moment. You can cheat and pop a mint into your mouth or take a sip of a drink.

This next stillness exercise can be conducted at work, perhaps at the nurses' station, and takes only a few moments.

EXERCISE 16.3   The Circle

1   Imagine a large circle on a piece of paper with a dot in the centre (you can actually draw this if you find it easier).
2   Take a few deep breaths, really focus on the dot in the centre of the circle, and inhale slowly.
3   Keep your focus on the dot, and hold your breath for a few moments.
4   Exhale slowly.
5   Repeat this process four more times.

Tip: A shortcut to stillness = roll the eyes upwards before starting the breathing technique, to initiate the alpha waves.

Chapter 16 Activity

Meditation often uses the assistance of nature to achieve a state of calm. This exercise may help to expel all the mental chatter in your mind to achieve stillness.

This beautiful lake is surrounded by pine trees and peace and calm. Take a moment or two to really look at the picture of the lake with its crystal-clear water.

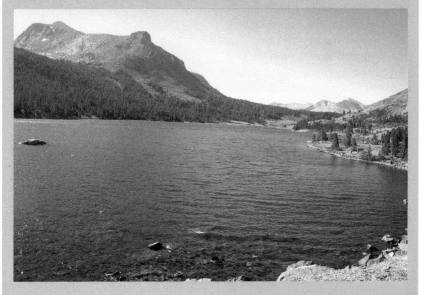

Lie down, making sure you are comfortable and will not be disturbed. Close your eyes.

Allow your body to melt into the floor or bed.

Focus your attention on your body and the gentle flowing of your breath in and out. Spend a little time experiencing the sense of your body as a whole, simply lying there and breathing.

When you feel ready, picture in your mind's eye the image of the lake in the picture at the start of this exercise. Imagine you can hear the gentle ripples on the calm, glass-like water, gently splashing against the edge of the lake. Imagine looking at the shadows on the water as the sun moves across the sky. Imagine how the light is reflected off the water in different ways – sparkling like diamonds.

Listen to the birds, and smell the fresh, clean air and the scent of the pine trees. Feel the gentle breeze on your skin.

Lie still for as long as you wish, soaking up this imagery.

KEY POINTS

- What is the stillness wellbeing technique?
- Practising stillness
- Benefits of practising stillness
- How to practice stillness
- Connecting with your senses
- Stillness exercises

WEB RESOURCES

Five senses stillness: https://www.mind.org.uk/information-support/tips-for-everyday-living/relaxation/relaxation-exercises

Stillness meditation: https://mindfulnessexercises.com/being-still-meditation

The power of stillness: https://psychcentral.com/blog/the-power-in-being-still-how-to-practice-stillness#

Benefits of practising stillness: https://makedapennycooke.com/10-benefits-of-practicing-stillness

PART 3
GUIDED MEDITATION FOR GROUPS AND INDIVIDUALS

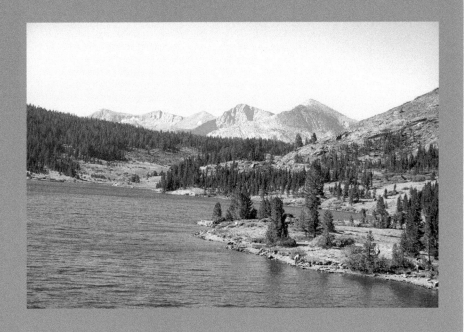

These sessions are designed for a group. I usually deliver them to small groups of 12 people in a room in the hospital where we will not be disturbed and no one can look into, so privacy is maintained throughout. It is always important for participants to feel safe and secure. I always mention that anything that happens in the room, stays in this room (think Vegas)!

Prior to the session, always speak to those wishing to attend to find out whether they have any allergies to the foods and essential oils that will be used during the session. Prepare a sign that states 'No entry', and put it in front of the room door. You may want to dress the room for a complete session, or just take parts from it: i.e. the visualisation script, if you want to do this on your own. All the sessions take the same format; they last about 40–50 minutes and have a fun activity incorporated. The scripts should be read very slowly, with pauses between sentences and appropriate music/sounds playing softly in the background.

Chapter 17
• • • • • • • • • • • • • • • • • •
SPRING

Cool Waters
Rainbow

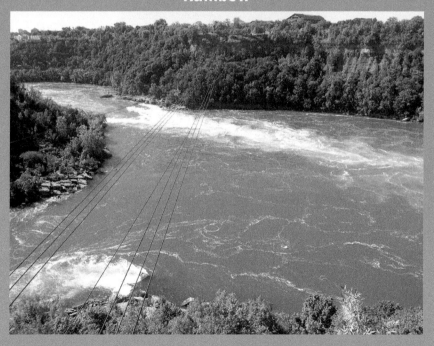

Wellbeing Strategies for Nurses, First Edition. Claire Boyd.

GUIDED MEDITATIONS SPRING

Cool Waters

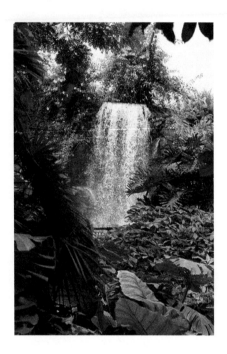

Participant pre-session information	For those wishing to attend, discuss allergies, etc. Ask participants to bring a yoga mat, cushion, and blanket and, for this session, a foot bowl and towel.
Room preparation	Place blue or white fairy lights around the room. If you are able, project pictures of waterfalls on walls around the room. Play relaxation music or sounds of waterfalls. Collect a bag of pebbles. Turn down the lights in room and close the blinds.
Essence of Cool Waters	Add about 12 drops of rosemary essential oil to your vaporiser to diffuse the room with scent. Rosemary oil is head-clearing and invigorating, perfect for the Cool Waters theme.
Food and drink	Lay out dishes of grapes, melons, and anything with a high water content. Prepare jugs of water with ice, cucumber, and mint, and cups. Have pieces of chocolate to practise eating mindfully at the end of the session.

Presents to take home   Prepare little bags of Epsom salts to put in baths to soak and relax.

SESSION

1   Welcome all participants and ask them to sit in the chairs provided.
2   Explain the importance of relaxation/stress for the body.
3   Ask the participants to fill their bowls with warm water (it is good to run this session quite near the bathrooms), and have them pour some of the stress relief bath soak (Radox is good and inexpensive).
4   Ask them to sit comfortably and put their feet into the bowl (after removing their shoes/socks, etc.). Some participants may wish to add a couple of pebbles to their water to feel beneath their feet. Get them to swirl the water around with their feet. They should enjoy the sensation.
5   After a while, having them keep their feet in the water, begin the diaphragmatic breathing technique from Chapter 4, Exercise 4.2.

When this is completed, have participants dry their feet, put the foot bowls to one side, and lie on a yoga mat with a cushion and a blanket, ready for the visualisation exercise. Participants may wish to put cucumber slices over their eyes.

MAIN SCRIPT

Get comfortable, either lying down or sitting in a chair.

Spend some moments scanning your body, which begins by slowly sensing the body in sections: feeling your feet . . . legs . . . hips . . . lower and upper body . . . arms . . . shoulders . . . neck . . . head **[see Chapter 13, Exercise 13.2]**.

Take a moment or two to focus on your breathing **[see the box-breathing technique in Chapter 12, Exercise 12.1]**:

Breathe in for four seconds.
Hold for four seconds.
Exhale for four seconds.
Hold for four seconds.
Repeat for six cycles.

Lie for a moment doing nothing. Let any anxious thoughts come to mind, and then let them go.

Now close your eyes if they are still open, and we will begin the visualisation session. Think of nothing but the colour black.

[PAUSE]

Now, imagine you are out for a long walk in nature. It is a beautiful, bright summer's day, and you feel the warm sun on your body.

Nature is all around you: visualise a lush green meadow of long green grass. If you listen carefully, you can hear the grass rustling in the slight breeze. The grass shines in the sunlight.

You make your way towards an ancient forest at the edge of the meadow, walking through the long grass. When you reach the edge of the forest, you breathe calmly . . . pure air, full of oxygen produced by the trees of the forest. With each breath, you relax more and more. You listen to the sounds of nature as you walk into the forest and the sound of the green leaves of the trees rustling in the breeze. It is relaxing, very relaxing.

You hear the sounds of the birds in the trees and smell the mossy forest floor, and relax more and more. You stop for a moment taking in all the beauty around you, the old centenary trees, their beautiful leaves . . ..

Now you hear the sound of water and walk towards it. You hear it getting closer and closer . . . it is calming, relaxing . . .. Then you see a waterfall in the distance and a beautiful pond.

Be aware of the rhythm of the cascading, flowing water . . . the water is crystal clear. You walk up to the edge of the pond and decide to step into the fresh, clear water. The water is cold on your feet and ankles. You feel all your worries melt away.

Next, you lie down in the water and float without making any movement. Spend a few moments floating as you listen to the waterfall in the distance. Everything is calm and relaxed.

[PAUSE for five minutes]

When you are ready, step out of the water. You feel refreshed and calm.

Slowly open your eyes and come back to the here and now. Perhaps have a little stretch.

Try to take with you this feeling of relaxation and calm.

End of session

At the end of the session, participants can eat and drink the snacks laid out for them. They may wish to eat some chocolate mindfully (see the activity in Chapter 13).

Give each participant their take-home present – a little bag of Epsom salts – and explain why this is beneficial (see Chapter 5, Exercise 5.6). Thank participants for coming.

GUIDED MEDITATIONS SPRING

Rainbow

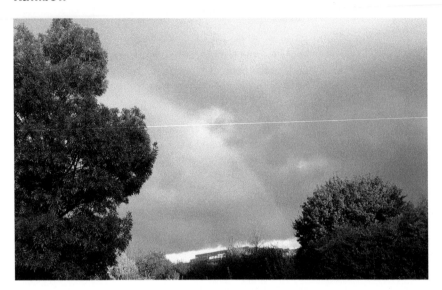

Participant pre-session information	For those wishing to attend, discuss allergies, etc. Ask participants to bring a yoga mat, cushion, and blanket.
Room preparation	Place coloured fairy lights around the room. If you are able, project pictures of rainbows on walls around the room. Play relaxation music. Blow up coloured balloons. Turn down the lights in the room, and close the blinds.
Essence of Rainbow	Add about 12 drops of sweet orange essential oil to your vaporiser to diffuse the room with scent. Orange oil is sweet and refreshing, perfect for the Rainbow theme.
Food and drink	Lay out dishes of fruits, incorporating all the colours of the rainbow: strawberries, blueberries, pineapple, peaches, kiwi, etc. Prepare jugs of water, cranberry juice, orange juice, and apple juice, and cups. Have pieces of chocolate to practise eating mindfully at the end of the session.
Presents to take home	Prepare little bags of Skittles for participants to take home (tasting the rainbow) and chocolate gold coins (to symbolise the crock of gold found at the end of rainbows).

SESSION

Welcome all participants, and ask them to sit in the chairs provided. Explain the importance of relaxation/ stress on the body.

Ask the participants to sit in a circle (on chairs or on the floor – whichever they are most comfortable with). For a bit of fun, play the balloon game: i.e. keep the balloons in the air and do not allow them to hit the floor (see Chapter 13, Exercise 13.3).

When they have finished this game, ask participants to sit quietly and begin the colour breathing exercise (see Chapter 8, Exercise 8.4).

When this is completed, have participants lie on a yoga mat with a cushion and a blanket, ready for the visualisation exercise.

MAIN SCRIPT

The first thing to do is to become conscious of your breath.

Inhale . . . and exhale. Inhale, feel the pure air fill your body, and exhale, feel your body release tension and stress. Again, feel the air fill your body and feel your body release all of the tension and stress.

Now we will begin the body scan exercise **[Chapter 13, Exercise 13.2]**.

Look for areas of tension, areas that cause pain. Visualise the breath filling the problem area, and on the out-breath, visualise all the tension and stress leaving your body. Feel the tension melt away.

Now we will begin the guided imagery.

Imagine stepping into a shower. But know that this time, the shower is magical. The water comes out at the perfect temperature. Just stand there and feel the warm water run over you. Keep your breathing relaxed, so it's nice and deep and slow.

The warm water has now washed away all stress and all tension. You look at your skin and see it sparkling with colour . . . like tiny jewels before it is absorbed into your skin . . . with all the healing properties. Look down at your feet, and see all your tension and stress being washed away.

[PAUSE]

And now the water starts to change colour. Firstly, the water turns into a beautiful vibrant red. The red water pours down and energises you right to your core. Just stand there a moment and feel yourself infused with the beautiful vibrant red. Feel this colour washing away all of your worries. They are simply washed down the drain and taken away. Now you are now free from worry.

[PAUSE]

After a moment, the water starts to change colour again, and this time, it becomes a brilliant shade of orange. Orange opens you to experience joy and allows you to release any feelings of guilt. Feel the orange wash over you. Feel the orange colour wash through you, washing away any guilt, and making more space for joy.

[PAUSE]

And then the water becomes a bright shade of yellow. Feel the yellow water cleanse emotional pain. Realise that some things are out of your control, and you can best handle them when you are calm and collected. Yellow clears the mind and invigorates. Take a nice deep breath and feel the clarity within.

[PAUSE]

Now the water turns to a brilliant shade of green . . . balancing and restoring the physical body. Green purifies the whole system. Feel the green water wash all over you.

[PAUSE]

Then the water changes to a beautiful, cooling sky blue. This blue enhances self-expression. Tilt your head back so that the blue water falls all over you. Let the warm water relax all the muscles.

[PAUSE]

The water changes colour again. It now changes to a colour containing indigo and purple. Feel it land on your head and wash all over you. Indigo and purple stimulate your healing power and wisdom. Indigo stimulates a feeling of calmness. Feel the calming influence of the dark velvet colours of indigo and purple.

[PAUSE]

And finally, the water turns to a brilliant glowing white light. Feel it embrace you, warm and pure. Take this moment to enjoy the white light that surrounds you . . . that fills you.

[PAUSE]

Enjoy how you feel. Enjoy being yourself. Know that you are perfect. And as you bathe in the white light, know that you are now cleansed inside and out. You are relaxed and calm.

Appreciate the last bit of this magical colour shower. Take a few refreshing breaths before you turn off the shower and step out of it.

As you towel yourself dry in your imagination, feel your body. Feel that your muscles are relaxed. Feel that your energy has been revitalised.

Become conscious of your breath. Wriggle your toes and fingers. Adjust your position, and slowly open your eyes. Sit up when you are ready.

End of session At the end of the session, participants can eat and drink the snacks laid out for them. They may wish to eat some chocolate mindfully (see the activity in Chapter 13).

Give each participant their take-home present: a little bag of Skittles. Thank participants for coming.

Chapter 18

SUMMER

Tropical Paradise
Summer Meadows

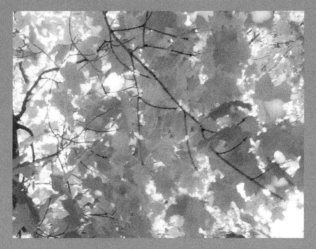

Wellbeing Strategies for Nurses, First Edition. Claire Boyd.

GUIDED MEDITATION SUMMER

Tropical Paradise

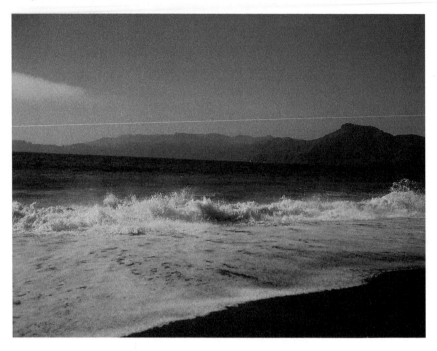

Participant pre-session information	For those wishing to attend, discuss allergies, etc. Ask participants to bring a yoga mat, cushion, and blanket.
Room preparation	Place fairy lights around the room – preferably ones with a tropical theme, such as pineapples, palm trees, etc. If you are able, project pictures of tropical beaches on walls around the room. Play relaxation music or sounds of waves. Place seashells all around the room. Buy mango and coconut body lotion. Turn down the lights in the room, and close the blinds.

Essence of Tropical Paradise — Add about 12 drops of ylang-ylang essential oil in your vaporiser to diffuse the room with scent. Ylang-ylang oil is intoxicating and warming, perfect for the Tropical Paradise theme.

Food and drink — Lay out dishes of mango, pineapple, and dried coconut (from health food shops). Prepare jugs of water and mango and pineapple juice, and cups. Have pieces of chocolate to practise eating mindfully at the end of the session.

Presents to take home — Prepare a bag with a little shell in it to give to participants at the end of the session. When they look at the shell, they will be reminded of the feeling of calm they experienced during this session.

SESSION — Welcome all participants, and ask them to sit in the chairs provided. Explain the importance of relaxation/stress for the body.

Have participants rub mango or coconut oil into their arms to evoke the smells of the tropics – place sheet with the lotion ingredients to make sure they are not allergic or sensitive to anything.

Begin the tropical island five-senses exercise **[see Chapter 14, Exercise 14.1]**.

Then begin the ocean breathing exercise **[see Chapter 4, Exercise 4.6]**.

When this is completed, have participants lie on a yoga mat with a cushion and a blanket, and begin the seaweed exercise **[see Chapter 14, Exercise 14.3]**.

Now get ready for the visualisation exercise.

MAIN SCRIPT — You will shortly experience a meditative journey, when you will be asked to close your eyes and allow yourself to be guided into a deep state of relaxation.

Keep your eyes open for a minute – don't try to control your thoughts. Think about subjects that come into your mind – don't fight them.

[PAUSE]

Now ensure that you are comfortable, and close your eyes. Review the thoughts you have just experienced. All the cares and concerns that came to you. What were the subjects and thoughts that came to mind?

[PAUSE]

Now, leave all this mental chatter behind. Draw a line under these thoughts. Remember, you are always in control – you can return to this mental state anytime you wish simply by opening your eyes.

I shall now count down from 10 to 1. As I count down, focus only on the numbers. As the numbers decrease, allow your thoughts to become increasingly calm – clear your mind, and become increasingly relaxed.

10, 9, 8, 7, 6, 5, 4, 3, 2, 1 . . . your mind is now calm, and you are feeling relaxed.

[PAUSE]

You are standing in a bright, white room. The floor is white marble, and the walls and ceiling are white. But you know that this is a safe place. You notice a door in this bright, white room, and you decide to open the door and cross the threshold.

[PUT ON DVD – SOUND OF WAVES]

[PAUSE]

You find yourself on a warm tropical beach with warm white sand beneath your feet, and palm trees. You walk across the warm white sand to a clearing in the trees and sit in cool shade. You are safe. The sun is high in the beautiful cloudless sky . . . beneath it is an aquamarine-coloured sea. This is your sanctuary. An island of happiness you have all to yourself.

After a while, you walk along the beach again and cool your feet in the warm surf. Take time to look around and feel the warm sea breeze on your face. Take in the experience with every one of your senses. Can you feel the warm touch of the sun? Can you smell the salty freshness of air? Can you feel the wetness of sand between your toes? Feel them all with your mind.

[PAUSE]

The beach is curved and surrounds the whole Island . . . continue your exploration by walking around the shore. As you walk, do you come across shells, corals, or rock pools?

The way you feel now is very different from the way you feel when you are stressed. Let the stress wash over you, like the waves of the ocean. Control your stress . . . diluting it with some of the calmness you feel now. You are able to recall the way you feel now. This is your antidote to stress.

Now look around your tropical Island for something that will remind you of this visit. Something to visualise in times of stress. An image, colour, object or feeling. Anything that will help you recall the way you are feeling now. Let your choice come naturally to you. Remember your choice when you next face stress in your day-to-day life.

On the beach in front of you, you notice footprints in the sand – are these your own? Yes. These are your footprints. You have walked right around the island by walking around the shoreline.

Go back to the palm trees, and sit and rest a while. We will now spend 10 minutes just relaxing and listening to the sounds of the waves.

[PAUSE 10 MINUTES]

You will shortly be leaving this tropical paradise.

Stand up and take a last look around your island, and bid farewell. You now need to depart.

Step through a hidden portal to the white room with the marble floor. Remember, you can return any time you want to this place of calm.

Prepare yourself to be awakened and brought back to the present. I shall count back from 10. By the time I reach 1, you will be fully awake.

[TURN OFF DVD]

10, 9, 8, 7, 6, 5, 4, 3, 2, 1.

Open your eyes. Your meditative journey is now complete. You may wish to keep still for a moment. Then wiggle your toes and fingers. Sit up when you are ready.

End of session

At the end of the session, participants can eat and drink the snacks laid out for them. They may wish to eat some chocolate mindfully (see the activity in Chapter 13). Give each participant their take-home present: a small shell to focus on and to take them back to this place of sanctuary in times of stress. Thank participants for coming.

GUIDED MEDITATION SUMMER

Summer Meadows

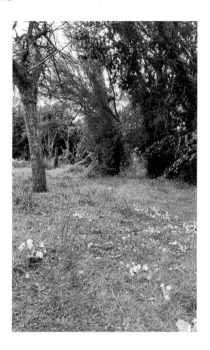

Participant pre-session information	For those wishing to attend, discuss allergies, etc. Ask participants to bring a yoga mat, cushion, and blanket.
Room preparation	Place coloured fairy lights around the room. If you are able, project pictures of flowers on walls around the room. Place flowers on the table – one for each of the participants. Play relaxation music, preferably something with nature sounds. Turn down the lights in the room, and close the blinds.
Essence of Summer Meadows	Add about 12 drops of geranium essential oil to your vaporiser to diffuse the room with scent. Geranium oil is piercingly sweet and uplifting, perfect for the Summer Meadows theme.
Food and drink	Lay out dishes of strawberries, raspberries, and peaches. Prepare jugs of water and elderflower cordial, and cups. Have pieces of chocolate to practise eating mindfully at the end of the session.

Presents to take home	Prepare compost pots and bulbs that participants can add to their compost when they get home so they can watch nature in action as the bulb flowers. Suggested bulbs include snowdrops or bluebells, depending on the time of year.
SESSION	Welcome all participants, and ask them to sit in the chairs provided. Explain the importance of relaxation/stress for the body.
	Ask the participants to sit comfortably, take a flower from the table, and begin the 'smelling flowers' breathing **[see the activity in Chapter 4]**.
	When participants are ready, begin the flower meditation **[see Chapter 12, Exercise 12.4]**, using one of the flowers brought to this session.
	When this is completed, have participants lie on the yoga mat with a cushion and a blanket, ready for the visualisation exercise.
MAIN SCRIPT	Lie down and get comfortable. You will not be disturbed. Close your eyes.
	You will shortly experience a meditative journey to a warm and safe place, and reach a deep state of relaxation. Don't try to control your thoughts in any way. Think about and acknowledge the thoughts that come to your mind. Think about these subjects, and then let them go.
	[PAUSE]
	During this guided imagery, you will need to follow my instructions as I guide you. Remember, you are safe. You are always in control. You can always return to an awakened state by simply opening your eyes. During the session, I will stop talking for 20 minutes, when you can enjoy the place I have taken you to in your imagination.
	I will count from 10 to 1. As I count down, focus on the number. As I decrease, allow your mind to become increasingly calm and relaxed. Here we go:
	10, 9, 8, 7, 6, 5, 4, 3, 2, 1.

[PUT ON DVD – NATURE SOUNDS]

Imagine you are the navigator of a canoe, guiding it down a river on a warm, sunny day. You are looking forward to reaching your destination – a destination all your own.

No need for haste – this place is always there for you. Ahead, you see a clearing on the edge of the riverbank. You know this is your own sanctuary. In a few moments, you will arrive.

After mooring your canoe, you walk up a short path. Here you find yourself on the edge of a beautiful field with flowers everywhere. The field is bathed in sunshine and surrounded by a lush green wood. No one else is aware of this place.

Find a place in the meadow where you would like to lie down. Feel the sun on your body. Enjoy being in this place of beauty. You are relaxed and at peace with the world around you.

Using all your senses, take in the whole atmosphere: the weather, the landscape, the plants, the wildlife, the smells and sounds. Take as long as you want in this special place of yours.

[PAUSE 20 MINUTES]

Be prepared. Lie quietly, and feel peace. The peace of belonging in such a land of beauty. Give yourself time to consider the things you are experiencing. Be reminded now of how you can manage stress. The way you feel now is very different from the destructive forces of stress. You can always control stress with some of the calmness you feel now. By being able to recall where you are now – you have an antidote to stress.

Now look around you and collect something to help dispel stress when you return: an image, colour, object, or feeling – anything that will help you recall the way you feel now. Let your choice come naturally to you. Remember this choice when you next feel stress in your day-to-day life. Conjure up this image.

It is almost dusk – the sun is setting. It will shortly be time to return home. Take a moment to watch the sunset. Try to capture in your mind the many rich colours you see: orange, red, yellow, gold, pink, and purple.

Walk back across the meadow. You see your canoe moored on the riverbank. Embark, and make your way back across the river. Take one last look back at the beautiful clearing. Remember, you can return to this place whenever you like. This is your special place.

With slow and confident strokes, you glide through the water.

Prepare yourself for your awakened state – back to the here and now. By the time I count to 10, you will be fully awake.

[TURN OFF MUSIC]

1, 2, 3, 4, 5, 6, 7, 8, 9, 10.

Open your eyes. Your meditative journey is completed. Wiggle your toes and fingers.

When you are ready, sit up.

End of session   At the end of the session, participants can eat and drink the snacks laid out for them. They may wish to eat some chocolate mindfully (see the activity in Chapter 13). Give each participant their take-home present: a compost pot and bulb. Thank participants for coming.

Chapter 19

· ·

AUTUMN

A Walk in the Forest
Moonlight

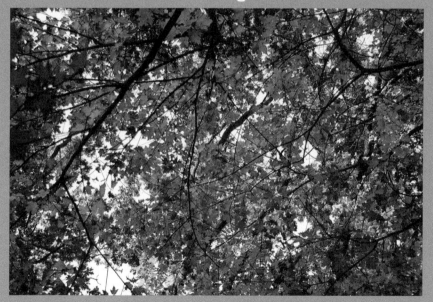

Wellbeing Strategies for Nurses, First Edition. Claire Boyd.

GUIDED MEDITATIONS AUTUMN

A Walk in the Forest

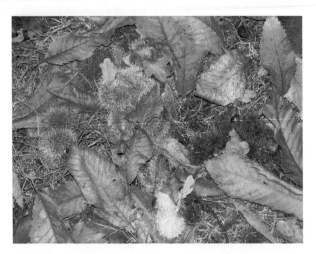

Participant pre-session information	For those wishing to attend, discuss allergies, etc. Ask participants to bring a yoga mat, cushion, and blanket and, for this session, water wipes.
Room preparation	Place golden-coloured fairy lights around the room. If you are able, project pictures of trees on walls around the room. Bring plastic bags, pine cones, and pine essential oil for the participant activity.
	Play relaxation music or sounds of the forest. Place an old sheet on the floor, and sprinkle on it leaves that have been washed and dried. Turn down the lights in the room, and close the blinds.
Essence of a Walk in the Forest	Add about 12 drops of pine essential oil to your vaporiser to diffuse the room with scent. Pine oil is cooling and enlivening, perfect for the Walk in the Forest theme.
Food and drink	Lay out dishes of fruit and nuts, such as blackberries (fruits of the forest), and blackberry juice. Prepare jugs of water and cups. Have pieces of chocolate to practise eating mindfully at the end of the session.
Presents to take home	Participants will take home a pine cone in a bag with pine essential oil.

SESSION

Welcome all participants, and ask them to sit in the chairs provided. Explain the importance of relaxation/stress for the body.

Ask the participants to walk on the dry leaves with their bare feet, feeling the leaves beneath their toes and enjoying the sensation of the crunch. Then have each participant put a damp pine cone (previously washed) into a plastic bag, and add 6–12 drops of pine essential oil. Seal the bag. After two days, this can be put in a room at home to benefit from the scent, and also as a reminder to take them back to the forest glade in times of stress.

After the activities, begin the humming bee breathing technique (see Chapter 4, Exercise 4.9).

When this is completed, have participants lie on a yoga mat with a cushion and a blanket, ready for the visualisation exercise.

MAIN SCRIPT

Begin by finding a comfortable position. Allow your body to begin to relax as you start to create a picture in your mind. Let the forest visualisation begin.

[PUT ON DVD – FOREST SOUNDS OR RELAXATION MUSIC]

Imagine yourself walking on a path through a forest. The path is soft beneath your shoes, a mixture of soil, fallen leaves, pine needles, and moss. As you walk, your body relaxes, and your mind clears more and more with each step you take.

[PAUSE]

Breathe in the fresh, cool air, filling your lungs completely. Now exhale. Breathe out all the air, feeling refreshed and revitalised.

Take another deep breath in – refreshed. And breathe out – revitalised. Your body feels even more relaxed.

[PAUSE]

Continue to breathe slowly and deeply as you walk through the forest.

The air is cool but comfortable. Sun filters through the trees, making a moving dappled pattern on the ground before you.

Listen to the sounds of the forest . . . birds singing. A gentle breeze blowing. The leaves on the trees shift and sway in the soft wind.

[PAUSE]

Your body relaxes more and more as you walk.

Continue to breathe slowly and deeply as you become more and more relaxed.

As you walk through the forest, feel your muscles relaxing and lengthening. As your arms swing in rhythm with your walking, they become loose, relaxed, and limp.

Feel your back relaxing as your spine lengthens and the muscles relax. Feel the tension leaving your body as you admire the scenery around you.

Your legs and lower body relax as well, feeling free and relaxed.

[PAUSE]

As you continue to walk through the forest, you begin to climb up a slight incline. You easily tread along smooth rocks on the path . . . feeling at one with nature.

[PAUSE]

The breeze continues to blow through the treetops, but you are sheltered on the path, and the air around you is calm.

Small saplings grow at the sides of the path.

Around you is an immense array of greens. Some of the leaves on the trees are a delicate, light green. Some leaves are deep, dark, true forest green.

Many trees have needles that look very soft and very green. The forest floor is a combination of thick, green moss and fallen autumn leaves.

[PAUSE]

Tall trees grow on either side of the path. Picture the variety of trees around you. Some have smooth, white bark. Others are darker, with coarse, heavy bark, deeply grooved. Enjoy the colours of the bark on the trees . . . white, brown, red, black . . . many combinations of colour. You admire the rough, brown bark of pine trees and enjoy the fresh pine scent.

Smell the forest around you. The air is fresh and filled with the scent of trees, soil, and crystal-clear streams.

[PAUSE]

Continue your forest walk.

You can hear the sound of water faintly in the distance . . . the gentle burbling sound of a small stream.

As you continue on your upward gradient on the forest path, you are getting closer to the sound of a running stream.

Continue to enjoy the forest around you.

[PAUSE]

You are aware that you can hear the stream very close now. The path curves up ahead. You can see sunlight streaming onto the path.

As you round the corner, you hear the water and see a clearing in the trees ahead. A beautiful lookout point awaits.

You are growing tired from your journey. Your body feels pleasantly tired and heavy.

Imagine yourself walking towards the clearing and the stream. Stepping stones make an easy path across the stream. Step on each large flat stone to easily cross the small, shallow stream.

Up ahead is a large, smooth rock . . . like a chair waiting for you to rest. The rock is placed perfectly, high up on this beautiful vantage point.

Sit or lie down on the rock if you wish. It is very comfortable. You feel very comfortable and at ease. The sun shines down on you.

[PAUSE]

You can look down from your vantage point into a valley with trees and a brilliant blue lake.

The clearing around you is made up of rocks, soil, pine needles, moss, grass, and bramble bushes, with lush blackberries ready for eating. The grass and bramble bushes around you blow gently in the breeze. A deer quietly emerges from the edge of the forest to graze in the clearing. As the deer raises its head to look at you, you can see its nostrils moving to catch your scent. The deer cautiously walks to the stream to drink before disappearing back into the forest.

[PAUSE]

Squirrels dart in and out of sight as they romp through the trees and race across the clearing. Soon they will be hibernating for the winter.

Feel the sun warming your body as you relax on the rock. Enjoy the majestic landscape around you, and feel your body relaxing even more.

Your body becomes very warm and very heavy.

Continue to breathe the clean, fresh air.

[PAUSE]

You feel so relaxed.

In unity with nature around you.

Enjoy the sights . . . sounds . . . and smells of the forest around you.

Feel the sun, warm on your skin.

Feel the gentle breeze blow across your cheek.

Listen to the birds singing.

Hear the stream flowing. The leaves rustling in the breeze. Squirrels chattering.

Lie back on the comfortable rock, and look up to see the blue sky. Small white clouds float gently across the sky. Watch them drift slowly by . . . shapes ever-changing.

Enjoy this peaceful place.

[PAUSE FOR 5 MINUTES]

When you are ready to leave this peaceful place, slowly begin to reawaken your body.

Know that you can return to this forest visualisation in your imagination whenever you like.

As you reawaken, keep with you the feeling of calm, peace, and relaxation.

[TURN OFF DVD]

Wiggle your fingers and toes to wake up your muscles.

Shrug your shoulders. Stretch if you want to.

When you are ready, open your eyes and return to full wakefulness, feeling alert and refreshed.

End of session

At the end of the session, participants can eat and drink the snacks laid out for them. They may wish to eat some chocolate mindfully (see the activity in Chapter 13).

Give each participant their take-home present: pine cones in a bag with essential oil. Tell participants to keep the cone in the bag for two days to allow the cone to absorb the scent fully. Thank participants for coming.

GUIDED MEDITATIONS AUTUMN

Moonlight

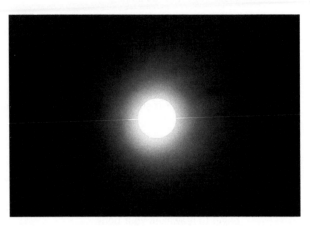

Participant pre-session information	For those wishing to attend, discuss allergies, etc. Ask participants to bring a yoga mat, cushion, and blanket.
Room preparation	Place round white fairy lights around the room. Hang Christmas baubles (white and round – moon shape) from the ceiling. If you are able, project pictures of the moon on walls around the room. Play relaxation music. Turn down the lights in the room, and close the blinds.
Essence of Moonlight	Add about 12 drops of lime essential oil in your vaporiser to diffuse the room with scent. Lime oil is cooling and awakening, perfect for the Moonlight theme.
Food and drink	Ask participants to bring a cheese to the session – something unusual, for the cheese-tasting exercise (see Chapter 13, Exercise 13.4). Bring cocktail sticks, crackers and grapes. Prepare jugs of water, cartons of red grape juice, and cups.
	Have pieces of chocolate to practise eating mindfully at the end of the session.
Presents to take home	Participants will make stress balls during the session.

SESSION

Welcome all participants, and ask them to sit in the chairs provided. Explain the importance of relaxation/ stress for the body.

Ask the participants to make stress balls using play dough and a balloon (see Chapter 15, Exercise 15.9).

When this is completed, have participants lie on a yoga mat with a cushion and a blanket, and begin the moon breathing exercise (see Chapter 4, Exercise 4.5).

Have participants find a comfortable position. Begin the PMR exercise (Chapter 5, Exercise 5.2).

Now get ready for the visualisation exercise.

MAIN SCRIPT

This starry sky relaxation is a guided imagery script that will describe relaxing at dusk and watching the stars appear in the night sky.

Continue to take slow, deep breaths.

As your body relaxes more and more, you can also relax your mind as you focus on the guided imagery.

Imagine that you are outdoors at dusk. It is still light out, but the sun has set below the horizon.

It is a pleasant temperature, comfortable . . . and you are in a safe, peaceful place in the open countryside, next to a beautiful pine forest. Picture this in your mind – calm, safe, and serene . . . a place where you would enjoy watching the starry sky at night.

[PAUSE]

Imagine the details of your surroundings. You lie on a blanket in the long grass next to the pine forest. Your position allows you to admire the sky above.

See the grass on the ground around you. Picture the trees next to the field of long grass where you are lying. Imagine this pleasant scene, and feel yourself relaxing, simply enjoying this solitude.

[PAUSE]

The sky is becoming gradually darker. The highest part of the sky is a deep indigo colour, becoming darker and darker as the moments pass. This colour blends into a lighter shade, almost green . . .. At the horizon, the sky is an interesting shade of pink, mixed with grey in the fading light.

[PAUSE]

It is very peaceful, watching the sky darken. The air around you is still and calm. In the distance, you can hear birds roosting for the night.

The air is slightly cooler now, very pleasantly cool against your forehead and cheeks.

[PAUSE]

Looking at the horizon now, shapes such as distant trees or buildings are in silhouette. Your eyes are slowly adjusting to the decreasing light. As you gaze up at the sky, it stretches from horizon to horizon like a vast dome. Straight up above, the sky is growing darker and is nearly black . . . fading to a lighter colour near the horizon in the west.

You can see the first stars appear . . . one star . . . and then another . . . and another . . .. See them twinkle . . . shining like tiny diamonds.

[PAUSE]

As you look at the darkening sky, you can see more and more stars.

Relax and enjoy the dusk . . . watching night begin.

[PAUSE]

The sky is even darker now. It has become a dark black, with only a slight hint of light at the horizon where the sun has set. The sky is so clear . . . you see no clouds anywhere to obscure the starry sky.

More stars have appeared, until the sky looks like it has been sprinkled by a salt shaker full of gleaming crystals of salt that are the stars. Some stars are bright, luminous . . . others are tiny specks that you can barely see.

Simply enjoy relaxing under the starry sky . . . enjoying this quiet retreat.

[PAUSE]

Now the sky is jet black. Out here, away from city lights, the stars are amazingly bright. Have you ever seen so many stars? The sky is filled with so many stars you would not even be able to count them.

See the constellations formed by stars . . . it is like hundreds of connect-the-dots pictures spread out before you. The starry sky is so huge . . . so vast . . . a beautiful glimmering blanket of stars stretching up in a complete circle around you from every horizon.

Admire the starry sky . . . feeling very calm . . . relaxed . . . at peace . . .

[LONG PAUSE]

Now it is time to leave this place. Slowly open your eyes. Stretch your body a little. When you are ready, sit up.

When your mind and body are fully awake, you can resume your usual activities, feeling refreshed.

End of session

At the end of the session, participants can enjoy the cheese-tasting exercise (see Chapter 13, Exercise 13.4). They may wish to eat some chocolate mindfully (see the activity in Chapter 13).

Give each participant their take-home present: their homemade stress balls. Thank participants for coming.

Chapter 20
· · · · · · · · · · · · · · · · · · · ·
WINTER

Candle Light
A Walk in the Snow

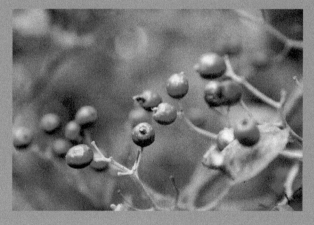

Wellbeing Strategies for Nurses, First Edition. Claire Boyd.
© 2023 John Wiley & Sons Ltd. Published 2023 by John Wiley & Sons Ltd.

GUIDED MEDITATIONS WINTER

Candle Light

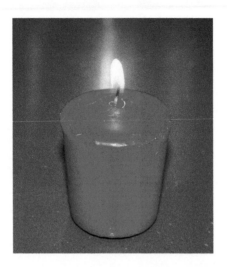

Participant pre-session information	For those wishing to attend, discuss allergies, etc. This session does not require yoga mats, pillows. or blankets.
Room preparation	Place electric tea lights around the room. If you are able, project pictures of candles on walls around the room. Print out pictures of a variety of candles and bring coloured pencils for the participant activity.
	Play relaxation music. Turn down the lights in the room, and close the blinds.
Essence of Candle Light	Add about 12 drops of lavender essential oil to your vaporiser to diffuse the room with scent. Lavender oil is calming and relaxing, perfect for the Candle Light theme.
Food and drink	Lay out dishes of 'happy foods': dried coconut, dried bananas, and mango and pineapple. Prepare jugs of water and cups. Have pieces of chocolate to practise eating mindfully at the end of the session.
Presents to take home	Each participant will take home two perfumed tea light candles.
SESSION	Welcome all participants, and ask them to sit in the chairs provided. This session does not involve lying down on yoga mats. Explain the importance of relaxation/stress for the body.

Ask the participants to colour in pictures of candles.

After this activity, begin the breath focus technique (see Chapter 4, Exercise 4.12).

Then begin the meditative session.

MAIN SCRIPT   To begin the candle visualisation relaxation, find a comfortable position.

We will begin with a body scan **[Chapter 13, Exercise 13.2]**.

Now focus again on your breathing.

Allow the tension to flow away as you breathe out.

Inhale as you raise your shoulders . . . then relax as you exhale, and lower your shoulders into a comfortable position.

Continue to breathe smoothly and gently.

As you rest peacefully, begin to form an image in your mind. Imagine that you are in a safe, comfortable room. The room is pleasantly dark.

Imagine the glow of a candle beside you. Keep your attention facing forward as you notice the gentle flickers of warm light on the wall in front of you. See the dancing light from the candle.

Feel yourself relaxing as you watch the beautiful patterns made by the light of the candle.

You might want to look at one of the electric candles, or choose to close your eyes and use your imagination.

Picture the candle in front of you, and see the soft light it creates.

Notice the flame gently moving as the candle burns.

Imagine what the candle looks like. What shape is it? What colour? What size? Create a picture of the candle in your mind.

Imagine that the candle gently melts away the stresses and tension you have been holding in your body. As the candle burns, feel the tension easing and relaxation flowing through your body.

Notice the wax becoming softer. Feel your body also becoming softer.

Notice again the soft flame at the top of the candle. See how it flickers slightly in response to your breath as you exhale. Watch how the flame responds each time you breathe.

Now turn your attention back to the wax of the candle. The softening wax is melting, turning to liquid. Warm and flowing . . . free from tension . . ..

See the wax of the candle melting . . . melting the way your tension is melting away.

As the melted wax builds, see it slowly overflow and pour down the side of the candle, drop by drop.

It feels like any stresses you were holding on to are dripping away with each drop of wax from the candle. The soft flame of relaxation warms you from the inside, melting away all stress.

Watch the wax melting . . . feeling the same effects on the tension in your body. Melting . . . relaxing.

Continue to observe the burning candle, enjoying the relaxation you are experiencing.

When you are ready to finish your relaxation session, take a deep breath . . . and exhale through your mouth, blowing out the candle.

Slowly bring your awareness back to the present.

Become more aware of the time and place you are in today.

Slowly stretch your muscles . . . and open your eyes . . . enjoying the feeling of calm and peace that remains with you.

End of session   At the end of the session, participants can eat and drink the snacks laid out for them. They may wish to eat some chocolate mindfully (see the activity in Chapter 13).

Give participants their take-home present: two perfumed tea light candles. Thank participants for coming.

GUIDED MEDITATIONS WINTER

A Walk in the Snow

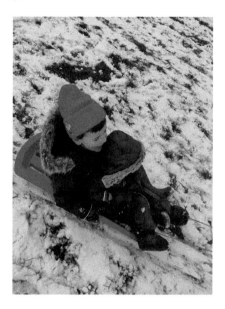

Participant pre-session information	For those wishing to attend, discuss allergies, etc. Ask participants to bring a yoga mat, cushion, and blanket and, for this session, their own mugs.
Room preparation	Place icicle fairy lights around the room. If you are able, project pictures of snowy scenes on walls around the room. Bring scissors for each participant and A4 white paper for the participant activity.
	Hang paper snowflakes from the ceiling. Play relaxation music or sounds of wind. Turn down the lights in the room, and close the blinds.
Essence of a Walk in the Snow	Add about 12 drops of peppermint essential oil to your vaporiser to diffuse the room with scent. Peppermint oil is uplifting and cooling, perfect for the Walk in the Snow theme.

Food and drink	Lay out dishes of strawberries and a chocolate fountain and skewers. Prepare jugs of water with ice, hot chocolate powder, and a kettle of hot water. If it's near Christmas, add a plate of mince pies. Have pieces of chocolate to practise eating mindfully at the end of the session.
Presents to take home	Little gingerbread men and women biscuits.
SESSION	Welcome all participants, and ask them to sit in the chairs provided. Explain the importance of relaxation/stress for the body.
	As an activity, participants will craft paper snowflakes (see Chapter 15, Exercise 15.12).
	When this activity has been completed, begin the cooling breath breathing technique (see Chapter 1, Exercise 1.4).
	Then undertake the `Melting the Ice Sculpture' meditation (see Chapter 1, Exercise 1.2).
	Ask participants to lie down on yoga mats, and begin the PMR exercise (see Chapter 5, Exercise 5.2).
	When this is completed, prepare participants for the visualisation exercise.
MAIN SCRIPT	Lie down in a comfortable position, or sit if you prefer.
	Close your eyes.
	Close your eyes. Let your breathing fall into a natural rhythm.
	Let your breathing fall into a natural rhythm.
	[PAUSE]
	Now we will begin the visualisation.
	You are walking through woodland blanketed by snow.

You are warmly wrapped up against the winter, and your boots crunch on the crisp, white snow glistening beneath you.

The air is crisp.

The sun is setting, dipping behind the tall trees, making the sky appear pink and navy blue.

The snow glitters on the bare branches like diamonds.

Your breath mists in the air.

The chill wind whispers amongst the branches.

Snow falls from the higher branches of the trees like stardust.

You are enjoying your walk in this winter wonderland.

You see animal footprints along the pathway – perhaps rabbits, foxes, and badgers.

[PAUSE]

In the distance, you hear a stream, a bubbling brook, cold and crystal clear.

Soon you come upon the bubbling brook and step on the stepping stones to get to the other side.

Soon the bubbling brook cannot be heard, and it falls into the far distance.

The tree branches begin to sway more forcibly in the stronger wind, and the sky becomes darker, harbingers of more snow to come.

[PAUSE]

As you continue your walk, you realise that there is no sound but the wind and your own footsteps.

This once-thriving woodland is quiet and frozen.

The scent of tree bark, fresh air, and earthy smells are pleasant to you.

Eventually, you come to the edge of the woods just as the snow begins to fall again.

Now you are clear of the woods. You quicken your walking pace as the wind becomes fiercer and the snow falls more strongly.

You turn up the collar of your coat as the sky turns even darker, producing gloom across the land.

Your cosy warm cottage lies just a short distance away, with a warm fire burning in the hearth.

Your feet sink more deeply into the snow, and the snowflakes hit your cheeks.

Soon you see your cottage and go through the gate and up the pathway to the front door.

Your cosy little cottage glows with warm, welcoming lights.

You open the front door, and warmth surrounds you.

You close the door behind you, take off your outer clothes and boots, and go into the main room.

You are glad to be home, as your legs feel tired and heavy, and you are ready to rest after your walk.

Candles are lit, lamps shine in a variety of colours, and fairy lights adorn the fire hearth.

Everything here says welcome and relax.

You draw the curtains against the darkness and the storm outside.

You stroll into the kitchen and make yourself a hot drink. Then you carry it back into the main room and sit in a comfortable soft chair.

As you sip your drink, you no longer mind the moan of the storm outside.

Here you are safe and warm.

Your cottage encases you with its peace and calm.

You smell the familiar scents that you adore.

You watch the flicker of the fire as the storm flickers outside.

But you are warm and cosy and safe.

You relax in complete contentment.

Soon you will go to your warm bed and a deep sleep, but all you need to do for now is feel the tranquillity of the moment.

Just listen to the wind.

Watch the flames dancing in the hearth.

You are completely relaxed.

[PAUSE FOR FIVE MINUTES]

When you are ready to leave this peaceful place, slowly begin to reawaken your body.

As you reawaken, keep with you the feeling of calm, peace, and relaxation.

Wiggle your fingers and toes to wake up your muscles.

Shrug your shoulders. Stretch if you want to.

When you are ready, open your eyes and return to full wakefulness, feeling alert and refreshed.

End of session At the end of the session, participants can eat and drink the snacks laid out for them. They may wish to eat some chocolate mindfully (see the activity in Chapter 13).

Give each participant the snowflake they made and a little gingerbread person biscuit. Thank participants for coming.

Answers to Activities

CHAPTER 6

Activity 6.1

1 Busy as a **bee**
2 **Pig** headed
3 Let the **cat** out of the bag
4 Open a can of **worms**
5 Going at a **snail's** pace
6 Hold your **horses**
7 The **lion's** share
8 One trick **pony**
9 **Elephant** in the room
10 Watching like a **hawk**
11 **Puppy** love
12 **Dog** eat **dog**
13 Let sleeping **dogs** lie
14 Wild **goose** chase
15 The world is your **oyster**
16 **Bull** in a china shop
17 A little **bird** told me
18 There are plenty more **fish** in the sea
19 Blind as a **bat**
20 Eager **beaver**

CHAPTER 8

Exercise 8.2

Idiom	Meaning
1. A red rag to a bull	Something that makes you angry
2. As brown as a berry	A person who is very suntanned
3. As white as a sheet/ghost	Looking pale and ill
4. Black sheep of the family	Someone who is different from the rest of the family
5. Browned off	Not happy about something

Idiom	Meaning
6. Caught red-handed	Catching someone doing something they shouldn't
7. Every cloud has a silver lining	Every difficult situation has a more hopeful aspect, although this may be difficult to see at the moment
8. In the pink	When someone is in good health
9. Once in a blue moon	A rare occurrence
10. Paint the town red	Going out and having a good time
11. Purple patch	A run of good luck/success
12. Red herring	Information that is intended to be misleading or distracting
13. Red letter day	A day that is noteworthy or memorable
14. Red tape	Something that often requires too much paperwork
15. The grass is always greener on the other side of the fence	A mindset that there is always something better in another place
16. Tickled pink	Being extremely pleased about something
17. Roll out the red carpet	To treat someone like royalty
18. Green thumb	Having a lot of talent for gardening
19. Got the green light	Getting the go signal to go ahead and do something
20. Green with envy	Extreme feeling of jealousy
21. Red in the face	May be due to embarrassment or being overheated
22. It was black and white	Straightforward, very clear
23. Golden opportunity	The perfect chance
24. Grey area	Something without a clear rule or answer
25. Rose-coloured glasses	Unrealistic view
26. White elephant	An expensive item that is costly to maintain
27. A bolt from the blue	Something that happens unexpectedly
28. The pot calling the kettle black	Classic example of being hypocritical
29. Blue blood	Denotes someone from a noble, aristocratic. or wealthy family
30. White lie	Telling a small lie that may seem justifiable to protect another person's feelings

CHAPTER 15

Chapter Activity

F	**O**	**R**	**E**	**S**	**T**	**B**	**A**	**T**	**H**	**I**	**N**	**G**		**G**	**R**
			O										U		R
			R					O							T
			T				M								S
E			H					U							A
X	**A**	**R**	**O**	**M**	**A**	**T**	**H**	**E**	**R**	**A**	**P**	**Y**			N
E	S		S	B	B										D
R	T		O		I	R									C
C	**H**	**R**	**O**	**M**	**O**	**T**	**H**	**E**	**R**	**A**	**P**	**Y**			R
I	E		N		P			A							A
S	S		I		H			T							F
E	S		A		I				H						T
			L	S	S	E	N	L	L	I	T	S			S
			I	**W**	**E**	**L**	**L**	**B**	**E**	**I**	**N**	**G**			G
R	**E**	**L**	**A**	**X**	**A**	**T**	**I**	**O**	**N**						G

Appendix A

· · · · · · · · · · · · · · · · · ·

EFFECTS OF STRESS

Wellbeing Strategies for Nurses, First Edition. Claire Boyd.
© 2023 John Wiley & Sons Ltd. Published 2023 by John Wiley & Sons Ltd.

Body

Increased heart rate
High blood pressure
Difficulty breathing
Difficulty swallowing
Feelings of nausea
Hyperventilation
Tense, contracted muscles
Backache
Immune system less efficient
Hot and cold flashes
Blushing
Sweating
Skin dryness
Rashes
Numbness
Tingling sensations
Increased blood sugar levels
Dilation of pupils
Dry mouth
Frequent urination

Thoughts

Difficulty concentrating
Difficulty making decisions
Frequent forgetfulness
Increased sensitivity to criticism
Distorted ideas
More rigid attitudes

Emotions

Anxiety (nervousness, tension, phobias, panic)
Depression (sadness, lowered self-esteem, apathy, fatigue)
Guilt and shame
Moodiness
Loneliness
Jealousy

Behaviour

Difficulty sleeping
Early awakening
Emotional Outbursts
Aggression
Overeating or loss of appetite
Excessive drinking
Excessive smoking or drug taking
Accident-proneness
Trembling
Avoidance of particular situations
Inactivity

Health

Coronary heart disease or stroke
Stomach ulcers, nausea, irritable bowel syndrome
Migraines and headaches
Asthma and hay fever
Skin rashes
Irregular menstruation
Diarrhoea
Cancer

Appendix B
COLOURING A RAINBOW

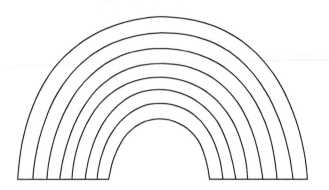

Appendix C

· · · · · · · · · · · · · · · · · ·

GLOSSARY OF THE PROPERTIES OF ESSENTIAL OILS

Property	Meaning
Analgesic	Relieves pain
Anti-anaemic	Relieves nausea and vomiting
Antidepressant	Helps alleviate depression
Antihemorrhagic	Helps stop bleeding
Anti-infectious	Counters infection
Anti-inflammatory	Helps alleviate infection
Antimicrobial	Resists or destroys pathogenic micro-organisms
Antineuralgic	Relieves or reduces nerve pain
Antirheumatic	Helps prevent or relieve rheumatism
Antisclerotic	Helps prevent the hardening of tissue
Antiscorbutic	A remedy for scurvy
Antiseptic	Destroys or prevents the development of microbes
Antiseborrheic	Helps control the production of sebum
Antispasmodic	Prevents or eases spasms or convulsions
Antitoxic	Counteracts the effects of poison
Antiviral	Inhibits the growth of a virus
Astringent	Causes the contraction of organic tissues
Aphrodisiac	Increases or stimulates sexual desire
Bactericidal	Destroys bacteria
Balsamic	A soothing medicine or application having the qualities of a balsam
Carminative	A sedative
Choleretic	Aids excretion of bile by the liver
Cicatrizant	Promotes healing by the formation of scar tissue
Cordial	A stimulant and tonic
Depurative	Helps combat impurity in the blood and organs
Deodorant	Corrects, masks, or removes unpleasant odours
Diaphoretic	Sudorific
Digestive	Promotes or aids the digestion of food
Diuretic	Aids the production of urine and promotes urination
Emmenagogue	Induces or assists menstruation
Euphoric	Causes a feeling of intense excitement and happiness

APPENDIX C: GLOSSARY OF THE PROPERTIES OF ESSENTIAL OILS

Property	Meaning
Febrifuge	Combats fear
Fungicidal	Prevents and combats fungal infection
Hemostatic	Arrests bleeding
Hepatic	Relating to the liver
Hypertensor	Raises blood pressure
Hypotensor	Lowers blood pressure
Insecticide	Repels insects
Nervine	Strengthens and tones the nerves and nervous system
Restorative	Helps strengthen and revive the body systems
Rubefacient	Causes redness of the skin
Regulator	Helps balance and regulate the functions of the body
Sedative	Reduces functional activity; calming
Stimulant	Quickens the physiological functions of the body
Stomachic	Digestive aid and tonic, improving appetite
Styptic	An astringent; stops or reduces external bleeding
Sudorific	Causes sweating
Tonic	Strengthens the whole or specific parts of the body
Vermifuge	Expels intestinal worms
Vulnerary	Helps heal wounds and sores by external application

Appendix D
· · · · · · · · · · · · · · · · · ·
WELLNESS BINGO

Cross off as many boxes as you can in a month. Remember to celebrate your achievements.

Eat some dark chocolate.	Meditate using stillness.	Go for a walk in nature.
Prepare a fruit smoothie using 'happy fruits'.	Use guided imagery to visualise a tropical island.	Take a warm bath in Epsom salts.
Keep a journal.	Wear a green top.	Do a three-minute exercise workout.
Dance like no one is watching.	Do some colour breathing (Exercise 8.4).	Read a book – one you have always meant to read.
Watch a funny movie or TV program.	Declutter your space.	Do a word search.
Hug a loved one or a tree!	Listen to soothing music.	Sniff some lavender from a tissue.
Bake some flapjacks, and invite friends over for coffee (or green tea).	Eat some fruit mindfully.	Do some crafting.
Do a couple of stretches.	Do the 4-7-8 breathing technique (Exercise 4.13).	Do a 'brain dump', write down all your worries, and rip up the sheet afterwards.

Index

Wellbeing Strategies for Nurses, First Edition. Claire Boyd.
© 2023 John Wiley & Sons Ltd. Published 2023 by John Wiley & Sons Ltd.